CRUSH CALORIES IN 20 MINUTES

CRUSH CALORIES IN 20 MINUTES

TRANSFORM YOUR BODY IN 20 MINUTES
WITH SIMPLE CALORIE COUNTED RECIPES,
WORKOUT & MINDSET HACKS

RICHARD KERRIGAN

NH
NEW
HOLLAND

DEDICATED TO MY DAD

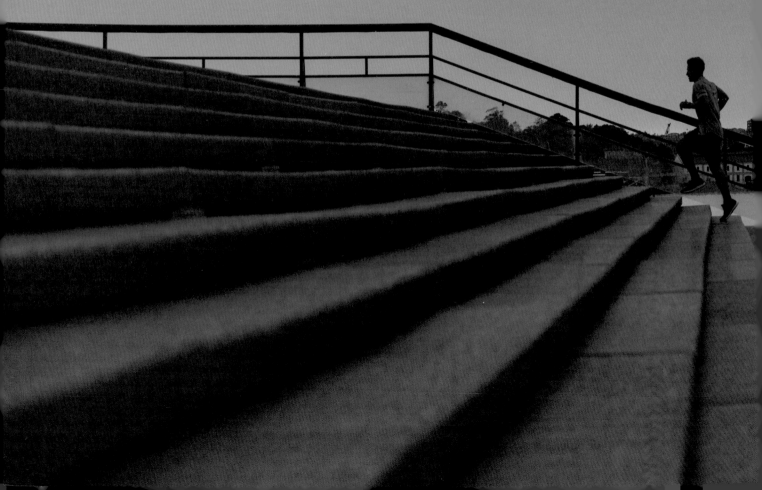

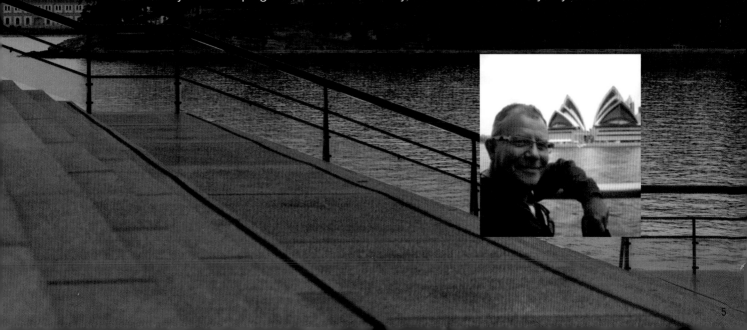

To my dad, who left us all too soon and is the main reason I work hard every day to ensure I get the most from this world.

Dad had a successful career as a television director and work was his life. He was always the first one on set and the last one to leave. However, the high-pressure environment demanded a lot and as a result the highs were very high and the lows extremely low.

In order to deal with the fast-paced lifestyle he would drink. He never had a hobby to allow himself to switch off, and there was nothing to steer his mind away from work. He said from as early as I can remember that he didn't have a problem with alcohol and I always believed him, right up until I started to witness first-hand some unforgettable situations where I knew he needed help.

I witnessed the alcohol consume him, impacting his health and then eventually taking his life. Dad passed away at the age of 61, still with so much life left to live. At first I was very angry for the wasted life, then as time passed I turned that anger into motivation, fueling my passion to help people live a healthy life and not to take their health for granted for one second; after all, without it we have nothing.

Food has always been a huge part of my life and I'm committed to helping people transform their lives through the power of food, simplifying the process to create delicious recipes that everyone can enjoy.

Dad: thank you for shaping me into who I am today, this book is in memory of you! x

Contents

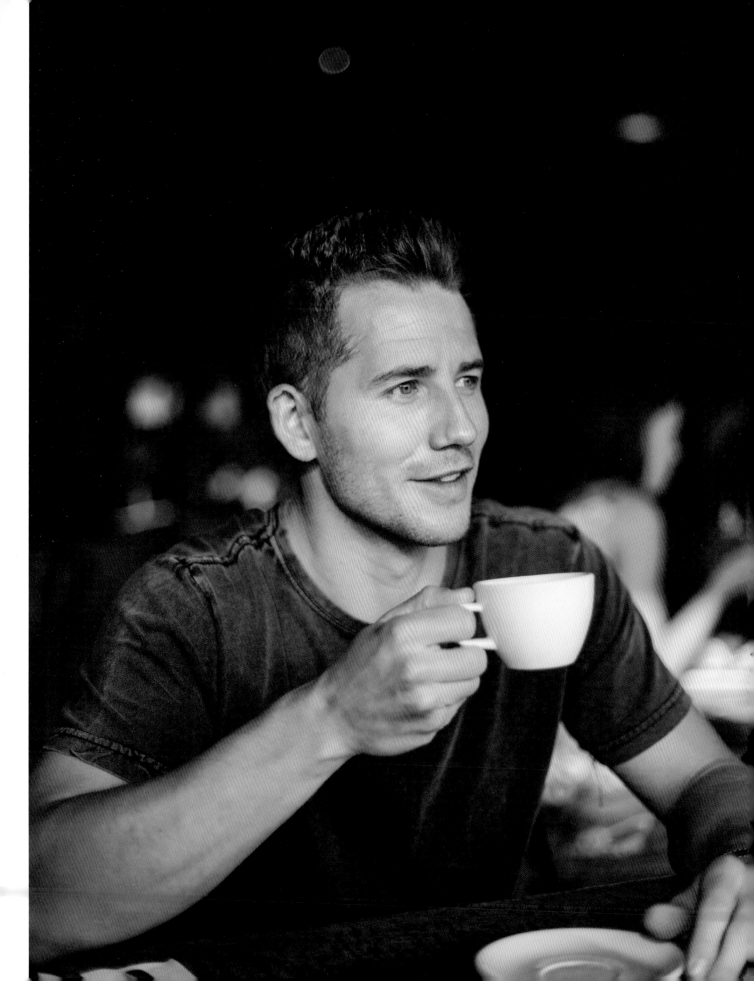

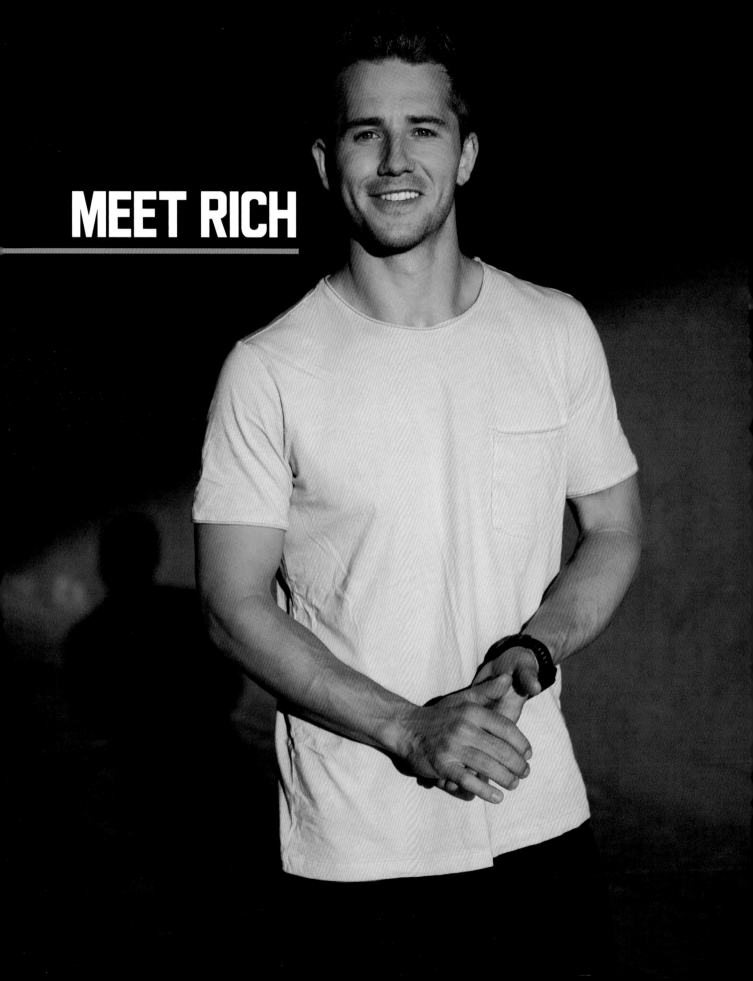

MEET RICH

My passion and love for food stems from my childhood. From as young as eight years old I can remember watching and helping Mum in the kitchen. I used to stand on a small chair as I could barely reach the kitchen top. I was fascinated by new, fresh ingredients and how easily you can create something really delicious.

Growing up, Jamie Oliver was my idol. I instantly connected with his passion and energy, he makes creating food look so simple and enjoyable.

As a trained chef and having worked in the fitness industry for 10 years, I'm now on a mission to show you that you can enjoy a healthy lifestyle that is sustainable, without feeling like you're missing out, or on a strict diet. I believe in eating real food that makes you feel good and is easy to prepare, leaving you to get on with your day.

I'm obsessed with staying fit and enjoy a whole range of sports. Some of my proudest fitness achievements to date are completing an Ironman in Cairns, Australia and also the New York marathon, missing the sub-three-hour mark by just 12 seconds (3:00:11).

I like to train my body through functional movement patterns, preparing it for life rather than for aesthetics, and I'm a big believer in playing the long game of health rather than relying on quick fixes which aren't sustainable and are way too restrictive.

After working with a broad range of clients over the last 10 years, I realized that the majority of people really don't understand how calories work and how they affect the body. If you want to lose weight you have to be in a calorie deficit otherwise you will just be wasting time and going round in circles.

I'm here to show you that you can create deliciously simple food and exercise at home or outside in just 20 minutes to help you crush those calories, lose weight and stay in shape forever! In this book I am going to share all of my secrets, training tips and lifestyle hacks with you, helping you to create a balanced sustainable lifestyle that you can enjoy for the rest of your life. It really is a great place to be when you are able to nourish your body with yummy food without feeling like you are constantly on a diet!

Food is there not only to provide your body with the energy you need to survive but also to make you feel good, which is such an important part of life. Once you build a healthy relationship with food – keeping in mind that *everything* can be enjoyed in moderation – you'll start to win!

There are 20-minute strength and cardio workouts that can be done at home with minimal equipment at the back of the book and you can find lots more time-efficient, super-effective workouts along with quick, calorie-counted cook-along videos on my YouTube channel **Richard Kerrigan**. And check out my website richardkerrigan.com.au and instagram page @richardkerrigan_ for more exciting content.

But enough about me let's get into the book …

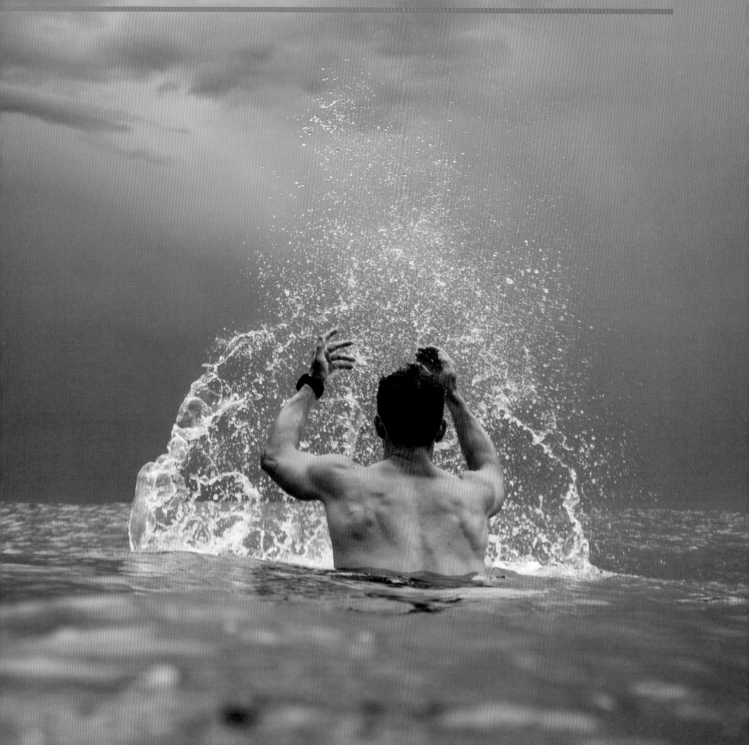

HOW CRUSH CALORIES
IN 20 MINUTES WORKS

*C*rush Calories in 20 Minutes is designed to transform your body in 20 minutes with calorie-counted recipes, workouts and mindset hacks.

There is nothing complicated about losing weight at all, yet so many of us struggle. Well not anymore! Now that you have this book, you'll learn the holy grail of weight loss that is so simple to understand and then implement, you'll be kicking yourself you've been wasting time on all those useless diets over the years. Oh, and speaking of time, this book is all about saving you just that … winning!

OK, I've left you in suspense for long enough, in order to lose weight and burn fat *you must be in a CALORIE DEFICIT*! It's as simple as that!

But counting calories can be painful and confusing I hear you say. Just relax because I've done all the hard work for you, clearly outlining the calories contained in every recipe in this book, leaving you with the simple task of choosing which delicious recipes you'd like to prepare in order to meet your daily calorie target.

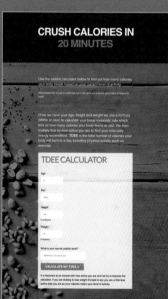

Now before you ask, 'But how do I know what my daily calorie target is?' I'm one step ahead of you on that. If you head over to my web page **https://richardkerrigan.com.au/calorie-calculator** you will see I have created an easy-to-use calorie calculator that will estimate your daily calorie needs based on your goal and current activity level, then come right back here and we can get cooking and start eating 'Go on off you go!'.

Now that you know your suggested daily calorie amount, it's time to check out the delicious recipes. In this book you'll understand how to portion-control correctly, how to eat to suit your body type whatever your goal, along with managing calories to fit seamlessly into everyday life. You'll find lots of other useful information on page 173 at the back of the book about calories and nutrition as well as tips for achieving long-lasting weight loss through calorie cycling – balancing your calorie intake across the week.

Simple Weight-Loss Tips Focus on these simple tips to help CRUSH your goal:

- Reduce your daily intake by 500 calories (if you were eating 3000 a day, reduce down to 2500)

- Increase your exercise slowly and focus on an activity you enjoy doing

- Build resistance training (weights) into your exercise routine three times a week

- Start preparing your food at home and limit eating out where possible

- Reduce your alcohol intake

- Drink more water, 2–2.5 litres (68–85 fl oz) is a great place to start

- Aim for 7–8 hours of sleep each night

Now onto my favorite part: FOOD!

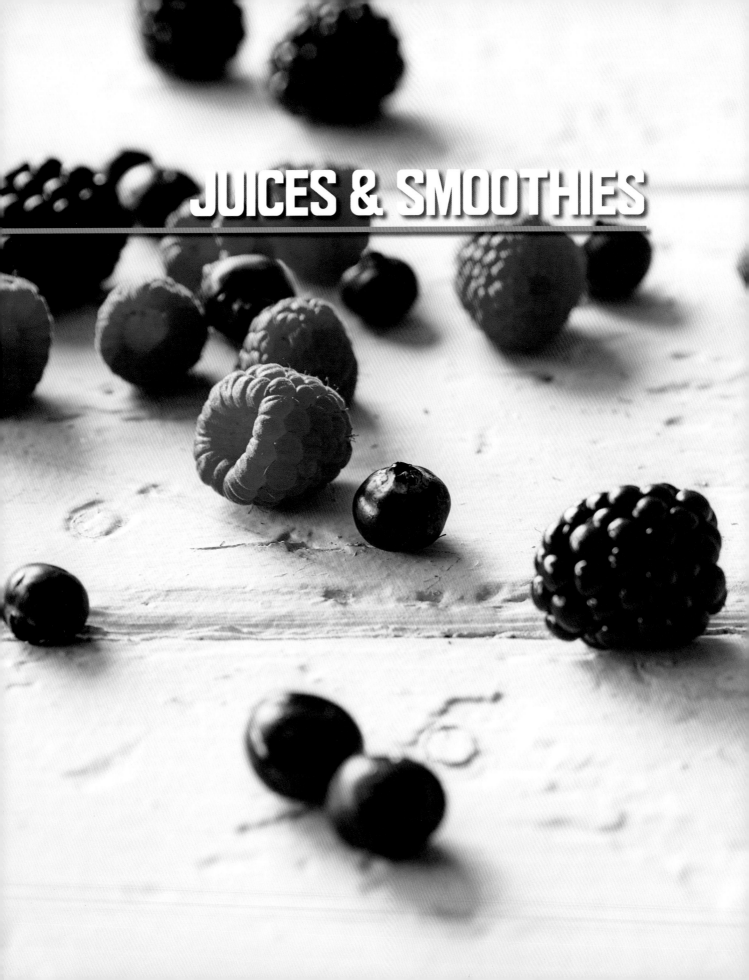

JUICES & SMOOTHIES

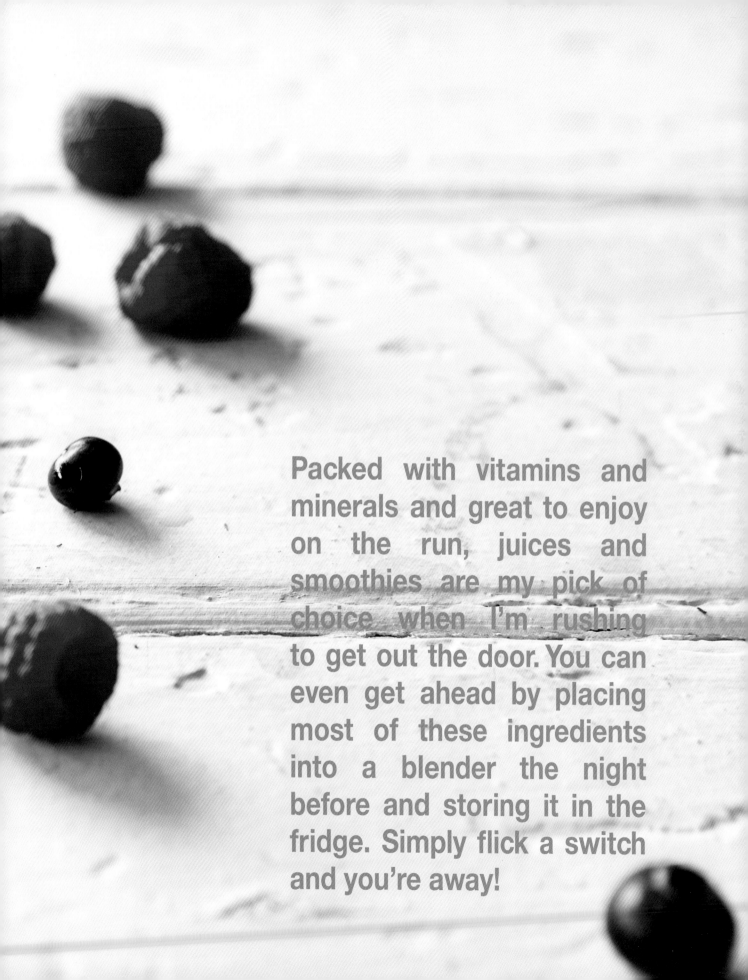

Packed with vitamins and minerals and great to enjoy on the run, juices and smoothies are my pick of choice when I'm rushing to get out the door. You can even get ahead by placing most of these ingredients into a blender the night before and storing it in the fridge. Simply flick a switch and you're away!

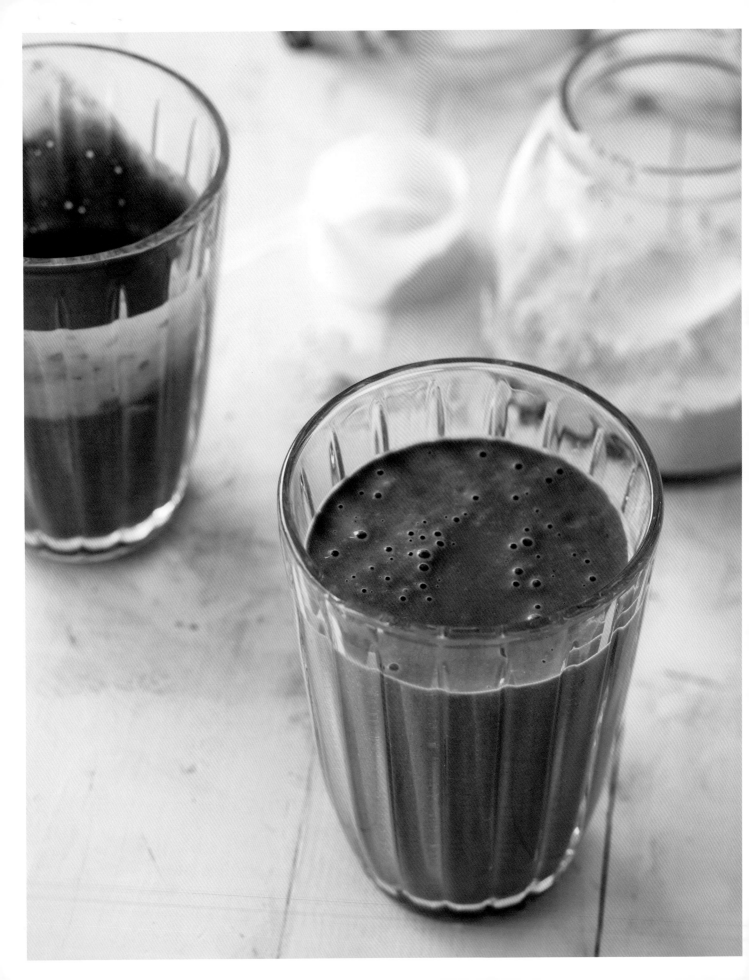

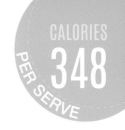
All recipes serve one.
Banana Rama

What better way to start your day than with a chocolatey protein-packed shake.
Just throw it in the blender and give it a good old blitz!

You will need:

1 frozen banana

2 tsp cacao powder

1 tsp peanut butter

30 g (1 oz) scoop of protein powder –

vanilla, chocolate or banana

1 cup of almond milk

lots of ice

Simple steps:

Put all the ingredients in a large blender, leaving plenty of space at the top, then stick the lid on and hit blend for 45 seconds. Enjoy straight away.

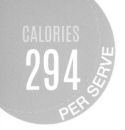

Brekkie Builder

I have this smoothie every morning without fail. It includes everything you need
to set you up for the day ahead and tastes absolutely delicious! #winning

You will need:

1 frozen banana

1 handful spinach

½ cup mixed frozen berries

cup pasteurized egg whites

1 cup almond milk

lots of ice

Simple steps:

Put all the ingredients in a large blender, leaving plenty of space at the top, then stick the lid on and hit blend for 45 seconds. Enjoy straight away.

TOP TIP:

Take a bunch of bananas, peel and slice in half, place into freezer bags and freeze ready for morning smoothies or homemade ice cream (see page 153 for banana ice cream).

GOOD TO KNOW:

As well as being a cracking source of energy, bananas contain a generous amount of **potassium** and they are also rich in **vitamin C.**

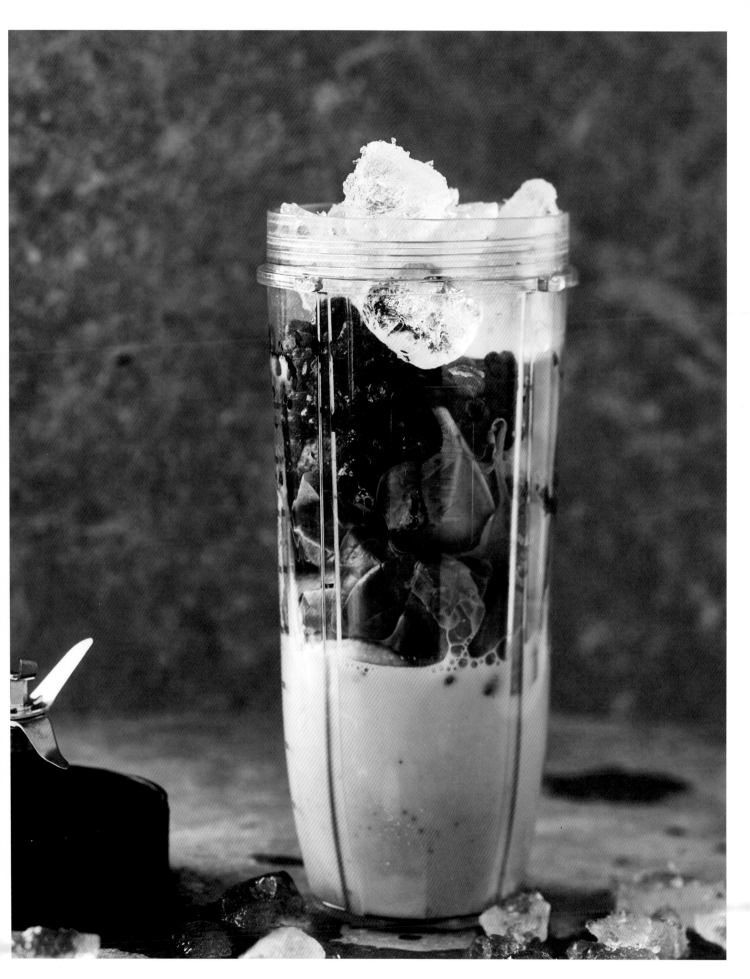

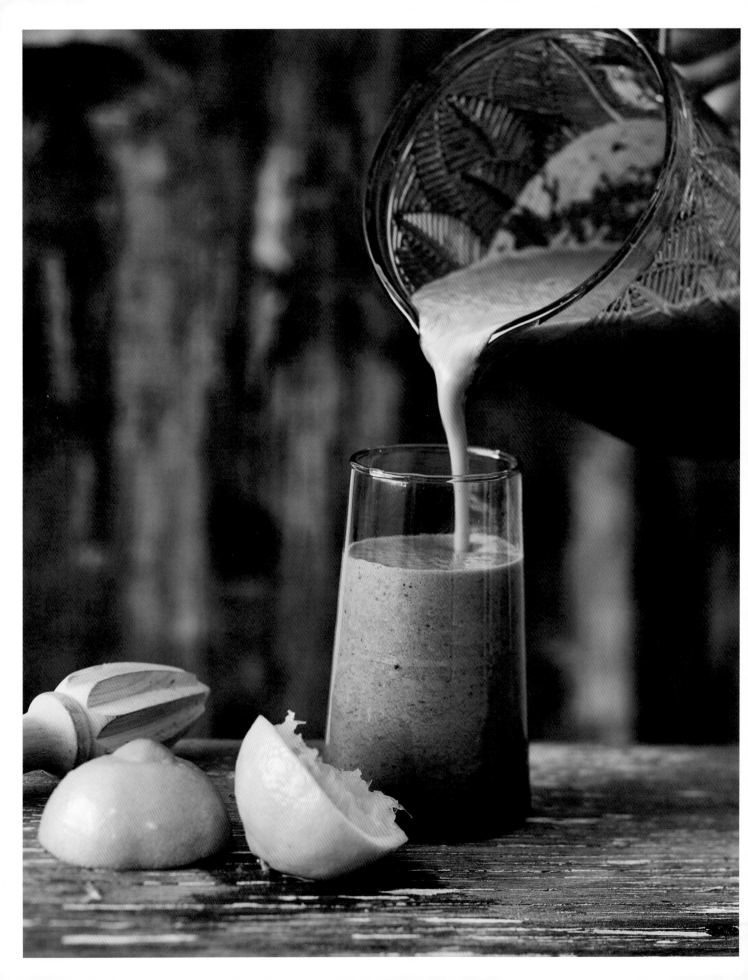

Lean and Green

Don't be fooled by the name; no raw kale was harmed or added to this juice.
I think you can agree with me that raw kale in a juice is like eating grass — yuck!
No, this lean and green juice is just full of yummy
good stuff that's really refreshing and super low in calories.

You will need:

1 stick celery
½ an apple, cored
1 handful spinach
1 cup coconut water
½ a lemon, juiced
lots of ice

Simple steps:

Put all the ingredients in a large blender, leaving plenty of space at the top, then stick the lid on and blend for 45 seconds. Enjoy straight away.

TOP TIP:

When you're making juices aim to stick to the 'two root (vegetables), one fruit' rule. This prevents you from consuming too much **fructose**, which is the natural sugar found in fruit.

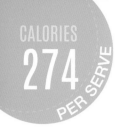

CALORIES
274
PER SERVE

Super Berry Blast

Mixed berries are my absolute favorite fruit to add to a smoothie as they deliver
super-sweet freshness along with bags of <u>vitamins and minerals</u>.
This is a great smoothie to make for the kids, with the calcium from the
Greek yoghurt helping to strengthen their bones.

You will need:

- 1 cup frozen mixed berries
- 1 handful spinach
- 1 tbs natural Greek yoghurt, full fat
- 1 cup cow's milk, full fat

Simple steps:

Put all the ingredients in a large blender, leaving
plenty of space at the top, then stick the lid on and
blend for 45 seconds. Enjoy straight away.

GOOD TO KNOW:

Mixed berries are packed with **vitamin C** and **vitamin K,** and because they are dark in color they are full of
antioxidants.

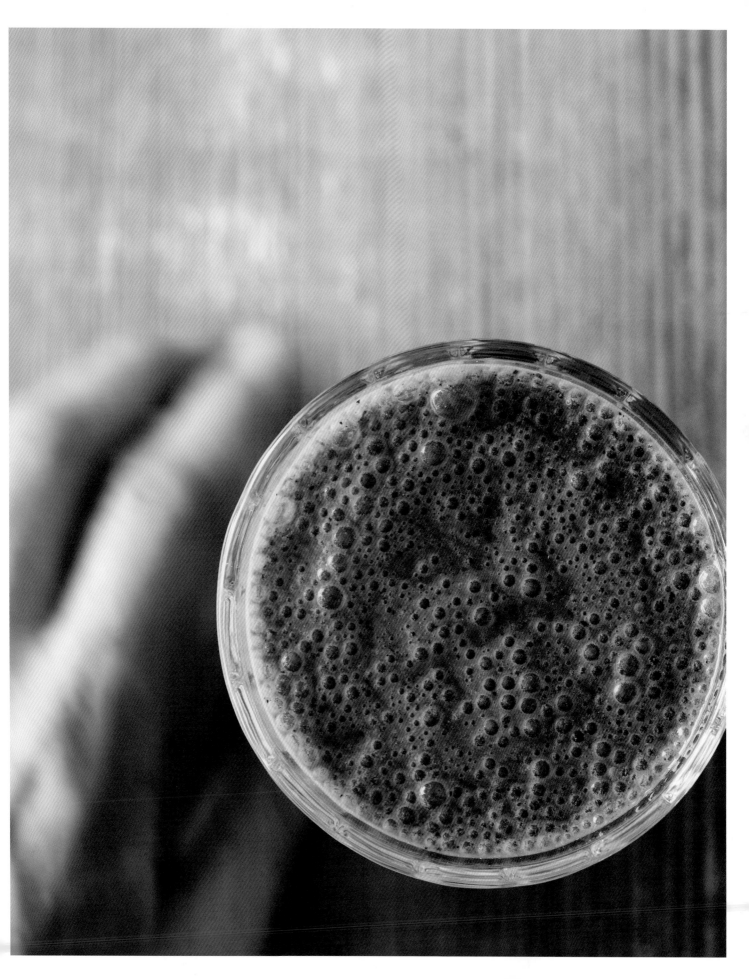

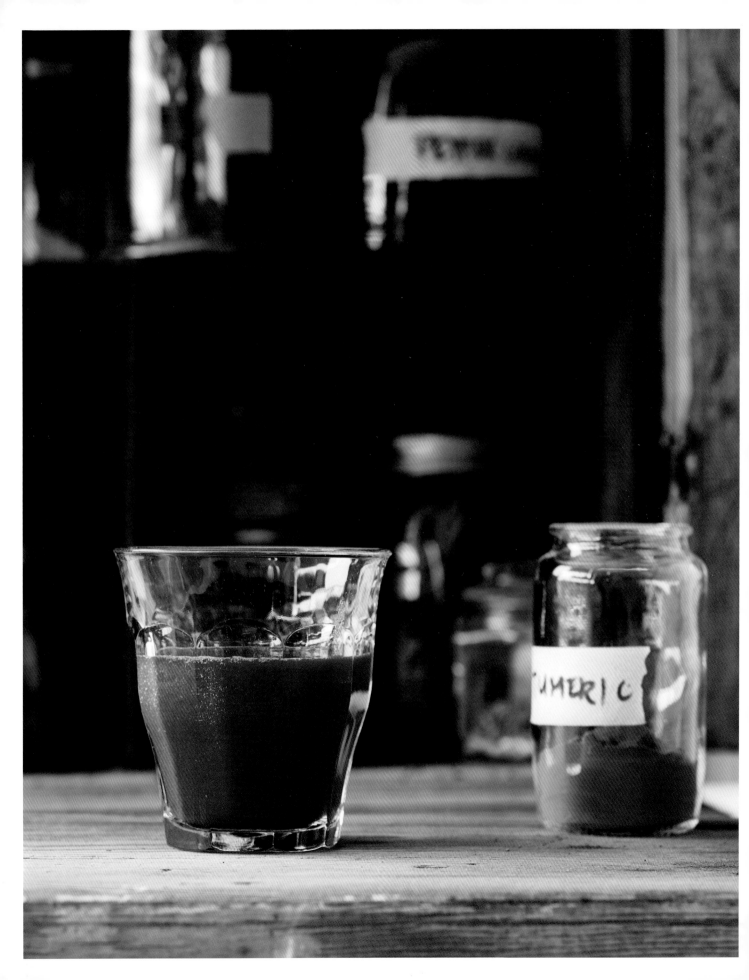

Beetroot & Turmeric Flu Shot

Beat the sniffles and energize your body at the same time with this delicious
flu-fighting shot. Ginger will help to wake you up while
the properties in turmeric are fantastic at helping with inflammatory issues.

You will need:

- 1 thumb-sized piece of ginger (peeled)
- 1 carrot chopped
- 1 cooked beetroot, sliced
- ½ a lemon, juiced
- 1 tbs honey
- 1 cup coconut water
- 1 tsp ground turmeric
- lots of ice

Simple steps:

Put all the ingredients in a large blender, leaving plenty of space at the top, then stick the lid on and blend for 45 seconds. Bottle the smoothie up and store in the fridge for a real morning wake-up. It will keep well for two to three days and the flavors will get more intense each day.

BREAKFAST

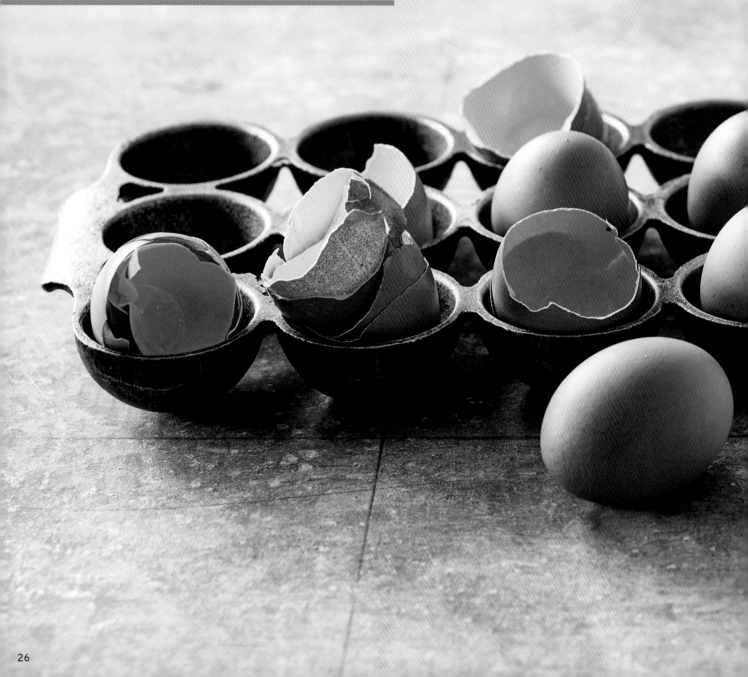

I'm a firm believer that breakfast is the most important meal of the day. However, I understand time is precious, particularly in the morning. That's why breakfast not only has to be nutritious in order to balance blood sugar levels, but also quick enough to prepare, leaving you to get on with your day ahead.

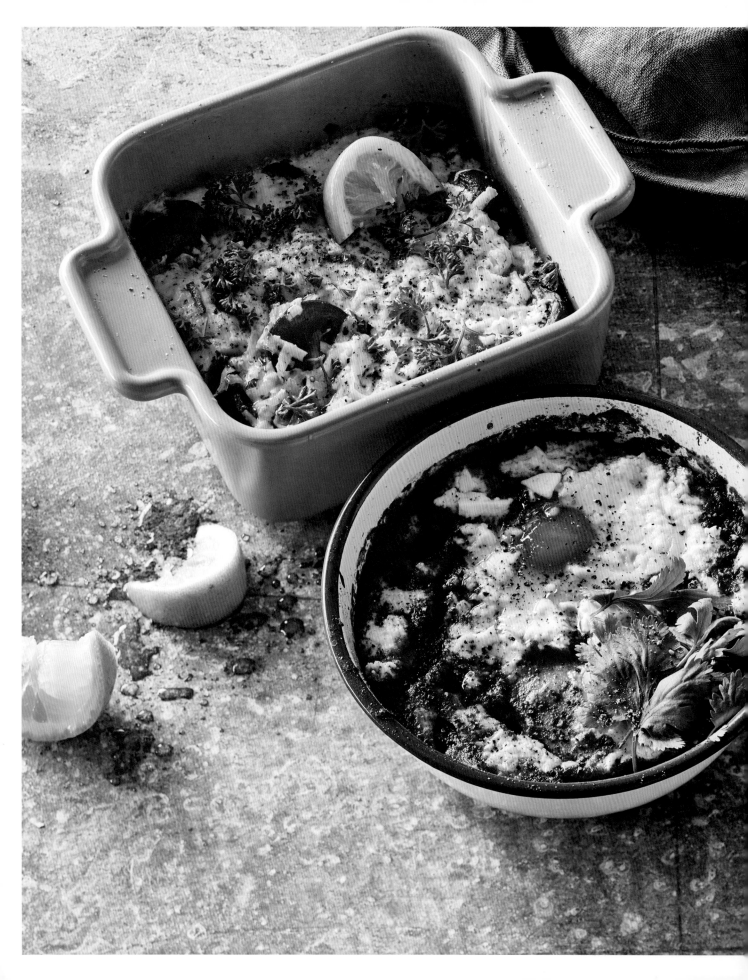

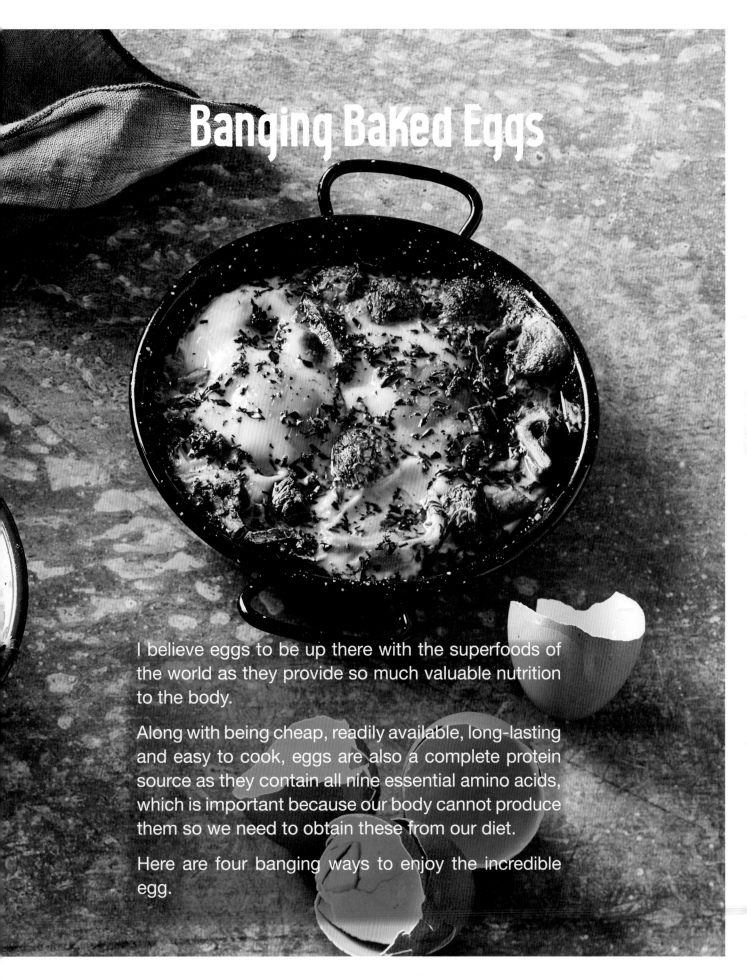

Banging Baked Eggs

I believe eggs to be up there with the superfoods of the world as they provide so much valuable nutrition to the body.

Along with being cheap, readily available, long-lasting and easy to cook, eggs are also a complete protein source as they contain all nine essential amino acids, which is important because our body cannot produce them so we need to obtain these from our diet.

Here are four banging ways to enjoy the incredible egg.

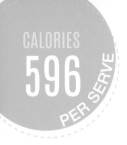

Greek Style

(SERVES 1)

You will need:

6–8 cherry tomatoes sliced in half

3 eggs

90 g (3 oz) halloumi cheese, grated

½ a lemon

¼ bunch parsley, finely chopped

extra virgin olive oil

salt and pepper

Simple steps:

Preheat the oven to 220°C/430°F. Drizzle a little olive oil into a small ovenproof dish and rub it around the bottom and sides. Add the tomatoes and season with a little salt and pepper.

Carefully crack the eggs into the dish and spread the grated halloumi over the top. Drizzle a little extra olive oil over the cheese and top with a pinch of pepper.

Bake in the oven for 15 minutes. Once cooked serve with a squeeze of fresh lemon juice and top with parsley. For best results serve with the yolks runny and enjoy immediately.

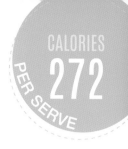

CALORIES
272
PER SERVE

Mushrooms and Thyme

(SERVES 1)

You will need:

6 button mushrooms, quartered

3 eggs

¼ bunch fresh thyme

1 handful spinach

extra virgin olive oil

salt and pepper

Simple steps:

Preheat the oven to 220°C (430°F). Drizzle a little olive oil into a small ovenproof dish and rub it around the bottom and sides. Add the spinach and mushrooms and season with a little salt and pepper.

Carefully crack the eggs into the dish and sprinkle with fresh thyme. Drizzle a little olive oil over the top and season with a pinch of salt and pepper. Bake in the oven for 12–15 minutes.

For best results, serve with the yolks runny and enjoy immediately.

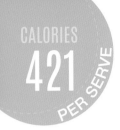

Shakshuka Style

(SERVES 1)

You will need:

1 garlic clove finely sliced

½ a red chilli, finely chopped

¼ bunch coriander (cilantro), leaves and stalks both finely chopped

1 tsp smoked paprika

1 tsp ground cumin

400 g (15 oz) tin chopped tomatoes

3 eggs

40 g (1.4 oz) feta cheese, crumbled

Simple steps:

Preheat the oven to 220°C (430°F). Heat an ovenproof pan over a medium heat. Drizzle a little olive oil into the pan then fry the garlic, chilli and coriander stalks until soft. Add the smoked paprika and cumin and fry for another minute. Add chopped tomatoes and reduce the heat.

Create three small pockets in the sauce and carefully crack an egg into each pocket. Crumble the feta cheese over the top then bake for 15 minutes. Once cooked top with coriander leaves.

For best results serve w ith the yolks runny and eat immediately.

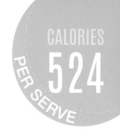

Middle Eastern Rolled Eggs

(SERVES 1)

Spice up your eggs and take them to another level with dukkah spice; it's nutty,
spicy and downright tasty when added to eggs.
This is one hearty breakfast you may even want to eat for lunch — and perhaps even dinner.

You will need:

½ an avocado

1 large tomato, sliced

a dash of white wine vinegar

2 super fresh eggs

2 tsp dukkah spice rub

extra virgin olive oil

1 slice wholegrain bread

salt and pepper

Simple steps:

Mash the avocado in a bowl with a fork, leaving a few chunks for texture. Season well with salt and pepper. Remove the eye of the tomato (stalk at the top) and slice into 4–5 even slices then leave to one side.

Heat a pan of water on the stove to a simmer, so you can see small rolling bubbles. Add a dash of white wine vinegar then crack an egg into a small cup and carefully tip the egg into the simmering water. Repeat with another egg then allow them to cook gently for 2–3 minutes. Once cooked, use a slotted spoon to carefully lift the eggs out of the water and onto a tea towel or a piece of kitchen paper to drain the excess water. Drizzle the eggs with a little olive oil and then roll them in some dukkah spice.

Pop the bread into the toaster then once toasted spread half the avocado onto the toast then lay the tomatoes on top, add a good twist of salt and pepper, finishing with the rest of the avocado. Sit the eggs on top of the avocado, finishing with a good drizzle of olive oil and a pinch of salt and pepper.

TOP TIP:

The fresher your eggs are, the better they will poach. When selecting your eggs from the supermarket or store, choose the ones from the back of the fridge or shelf.

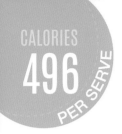

Chocolate and Berry Overnight Oats

(SERVES 2)

Preparing these simple overnight oats leaves you with virtually nothing to do in the morning.
Simply remove the cover and dunk your spoon straight in.

You will need:

1 cup porridge oats

¼ cup chia seeds

2 tsp ground cinnamon

2 tsp honey

2 tbs full fat natural yoghurt

1 ½ cups almond milk

2 tsp cacao powder

1 ½ cups frozen mixed berries

cacao nibs to top

Simple steps:

Put the oats, cacao powder, chia seeds, cinnamon, honey, 1 tablespoon of yoghurt and the almond milk in a bowl and give it a good stir. Put Add the frozen berries in to a small non-metallic bowl and stick them in the microwave for 45 seconds on defrost. Using a fork mash the berries up a little then add to the oats.

Grab two clean jam jars or large glasses and spoon in the oats. Cover each one and store in the fridge overnight. In the morning top each one with half a spoon of natural yoghurt and a sprinkling of cacao nibs.

TOP TIP:

Another win is these little breakfast pots will keep really well in the fridge for up to three days.

GOOD TO KNOW:

Porridge oats provide **slow-releasing energy,** keeping your blood sugars level. Along with being a great source of polyunsaturated fat and omega 3s, chia seeds are a good source of dietary fiber.

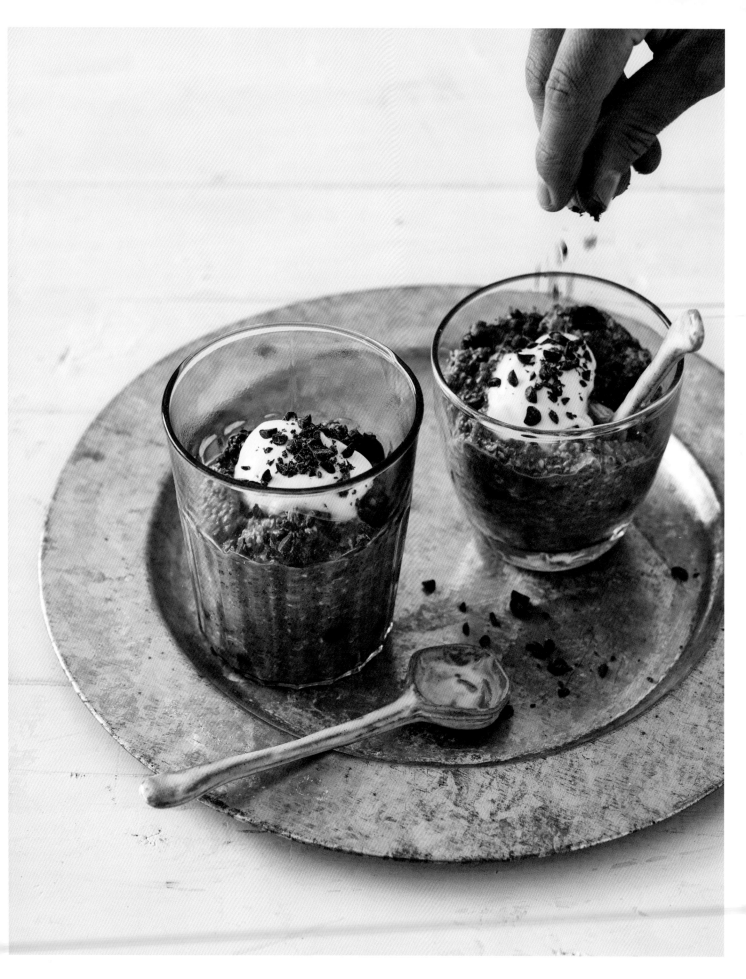

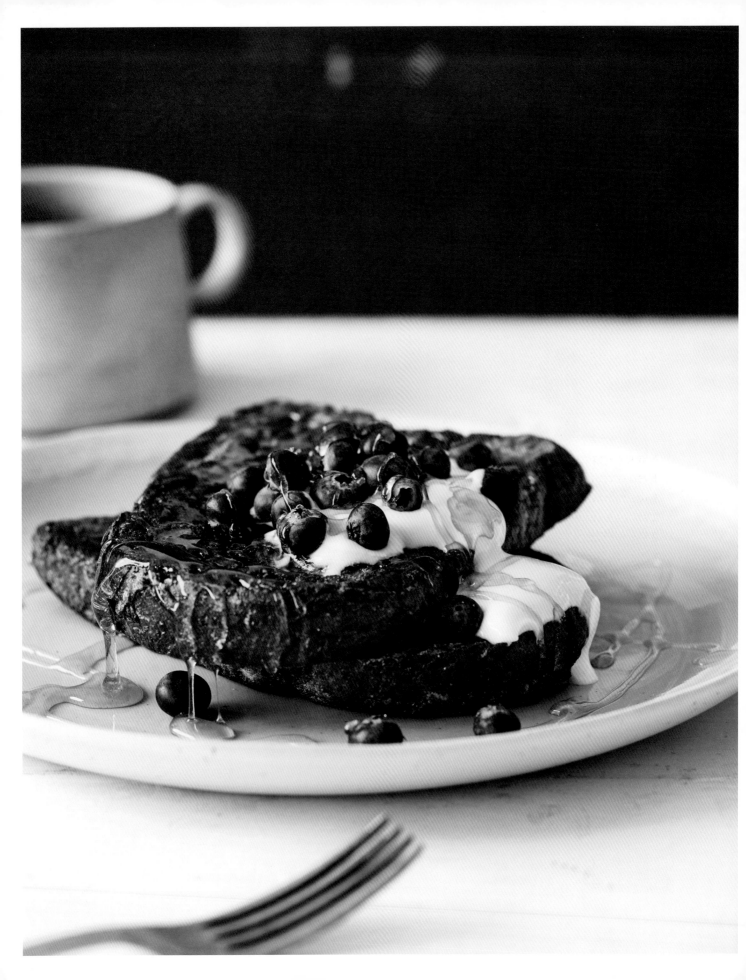

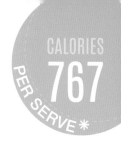

OMG French Toast

(SERVES 1)

Elevate boring eggy bread with sweet maple syrup, tangy yoghurt and fresh blueberries.
Yes, ok so it's a little on the indulgent side, but hey, life's all about balance right?!
Trust me you'll be making this again and again, I just know it.

You will need:

- 3 large eggs
- 1 tsp ground cinnamon
- 1 tbs maple syrup or honey
- 2 slices wholemeal bread
- 2 tbs full fat natural yoghurt
- 1 handful blueberries
- 2 tbs extra virgin olive oil

Simple steps:

Whisk the eggs in a large bowl with a fork and add the cinnamon and maple syrup.

Dip the bread into the egg and coat well, flipping it over several times to ensure the egg is well soaked into the bread.

Heat a non-stick pan over a medium heat with a light drizzle of olive oil. Once hot carefully place the eggy bread into the pan and spoon any leftover egg onto the bread. Fry for 60–90 seconds then carefully flip over. Serve the toast with yoghurt and blueberries. Finish with an extra drizzle of maple syrup.

* Need this recipe a little lighter?
Simply reduce the olive oil 1 tbs (20ml) olive oil = 165 calories

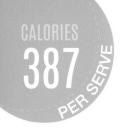
Funky Fungi Omelet

(SERVES 1)

Omelets are a delicious way to enjoy eggs, and the combinations really are endless.
The hard part was trying to pick a favorite, but there's just something
about mushrooms and fresh tarragon that make this my number-one combo.

You will need:

2 handfuls exotic mushrooms, sliced

1 garlic clove, finely chopped

¼ bunch fresh tarragon, roughly chopped

2 handfuls spinach

3 eggs

extra virgin olive oil

salt and pepper

Simple steps:

Pan fry the mushrooms and garlic in a non-stick pan with a little olive oil over a medium heat, seasoning with a pinch of salt and pepper. Your aim here is to draw out as much of the water from the mushrooms as possible. After 2–3 minutes add the fresh tarragon. Add the spinach and allow it to soften. Once soft transfer the mushrooms and spinach to a small bowl. Wipe the pan clean and add a little extra olive oil.

Whisk the eggs in a small bowl, season with a pinch of salt and pepper then add to the pan. Stir and move the eggs around the pan so they cook quickly and evenly. Add the mushrooms and spinach to one half of the omelet then carefully fold the other half over the top. Slide onto a plate and serve with a twist of black pepper.

TOP TIP:

Omelets actually reheat really well. So, if you exercise first thing in the morning then head straight to the office, simply make this the night before and reheat in the microwave at work. Cook it a little soft so when you reheat it, it doesn't dry out.

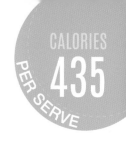

CALORIES
435
PER SERVE

Exotic Mushies and Zucchini Eggs Straight from the Pan

(SERVES 2)

Now your mum would probably tell you off for eating straight from the pan, but this really is the only way to eat this yummy breakfast. This is my lazy Sunday morning feast when I just want to sit back, relax and take it slow.

You will need:

150 g (5 oz) exotic mushrooms, sliced

1/2 brown onion, finely diced

1 garlic clove, finely chopped

1 large zucchini, sliced

1/2 bunch thyme

3 large handfuls spinach

4 eggs

½ tsp chilli flakes

60 g (2 oz) parmesan cheese

extra virgin olive oil

salt and pepper

Simple steps:

Wash the mushrooms well and dry with some kitchen paper. Slice the mushrooms so they are all roughly the same size then leave to one side.

Pan fry the onion and garlic in a little olive oil until soft. Add the mushrooms, zucchini and fresh thyme along with a good pinch of salt and pepper and fry for 2–3 minutes. Add the spinach and give the pan a good toss. Place a lid on the pan, remove from the heat and leave to one side. This will allow the spinach to soften.

Preheat the grill. In a separate pan, fry two eggs in a little oil over a medium heat. Once cooked, place the eggs on top of the mushrooms while they are still in the pan, and sprinkle a few chilli flakes over the top. Repeat with remaining eggs. Shave parmesan cheese over the top and place the pan under the grill for 90 seconds.

Place the pan in the middle of the table and serve immediately with a side of toast and a fresh pot of coffee. Heaven!

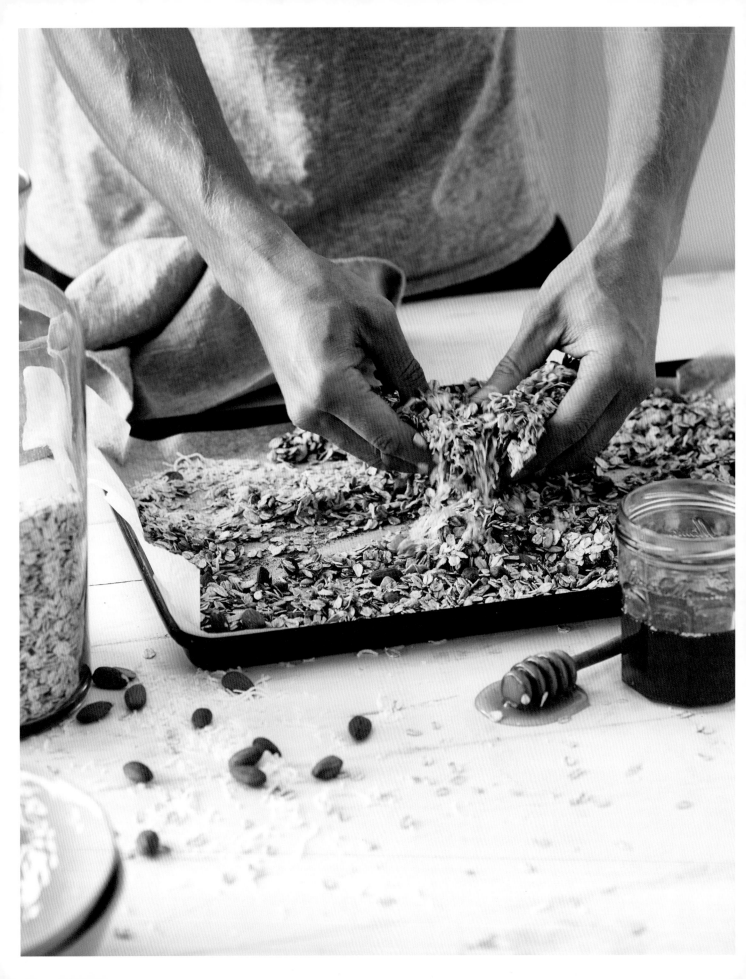

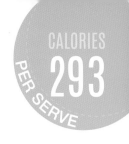

Mum's 'Too Good' Toasted Granola

(10 SERVINGS)

My mum used to make this for my sister and I growing up, and we would always
have a large jar of it in the cupboard at home. Not only is it great to
kickstart the day, but I love sprinkling it on top of some fruit or even adding
it to a smoothie to provide a little energy boost.

You will need:

- 3 cups porridge oats
- ½ cup almonds, roughly chopped
- ½ cup sunflower seeds
- 4 tsp ground cinnamon
- ½ cup flax seeds
- 3 tbs rice bran syrup
- ½ cup coconut shavings
- pinch of sea salt

Simple steps:

Preheat your oven to 180°C (350°F). Line a large tray with a sheet of baking paper.

In a large bowl mix the oats, almonds, sunflower seeds, cinnamon, flax seeds and a pinch of salt. Spread evenly on the tray – use two trays if necessary as you want the mix to be spread thinly. Drizzle the rice bran syrup over the top then toast in the oven for 10 minutes. Remove from the oven then toss the oats around so the oats at the bottom are now at the top. Return to the oven for another 5 minutes.

Once toasted add the coconut shavings and leave to cool. Store in a large airtight jar in the cupboard.

GOOD TO KNOW:

Cinnamon is a great source of **fiber** and also contains antioxidant properties, helping us to stay healthy and age well.

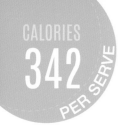
Chilli Tomato Frittata

(SERVES 4)

Weekend wake-ups just got a whole lot better!
This super-charged omelette, baked and served in the pan, straight from the oven,
is definitely one for sharing. Place it in the middle of the breakfast table and just dig in.

You will need:

½ a white onion, finely diced

10–12 sun-dried tomatoes, roughly chopped

3 large handfuls spinach

8–10 eggs

1 tsp chilli flakes

1 bunch asparagus spears

100 g (3 ½ oz) parmesan cheese

½ a lemon, juiced

extra virgin olive oil

salt and pepper

Simple steps:

Preheat your oven to 200°C (350°F). Heat a large ovenproof pan and drizzle with a little olive oil. Pan fry the onions until soft. Add the sun-dried tomatoes and spinach and allow to soften.

Whisk the eggs in a large bowl, seasoning with salt, pepper and chilli flakes, then add to the pan. Stir for a minute to speed up the cooking. Cut about 3 cm (1 in) off the end of the asparagus spears and discard. Slice the spears in half lengthways then add to the eggs. Grate the parmesan cheese over the top then place the pan in the oven and bake for 12–15 minutes. Serve straight from the pan with some extra chill flakes on top and a squeeze of fresh lemon.

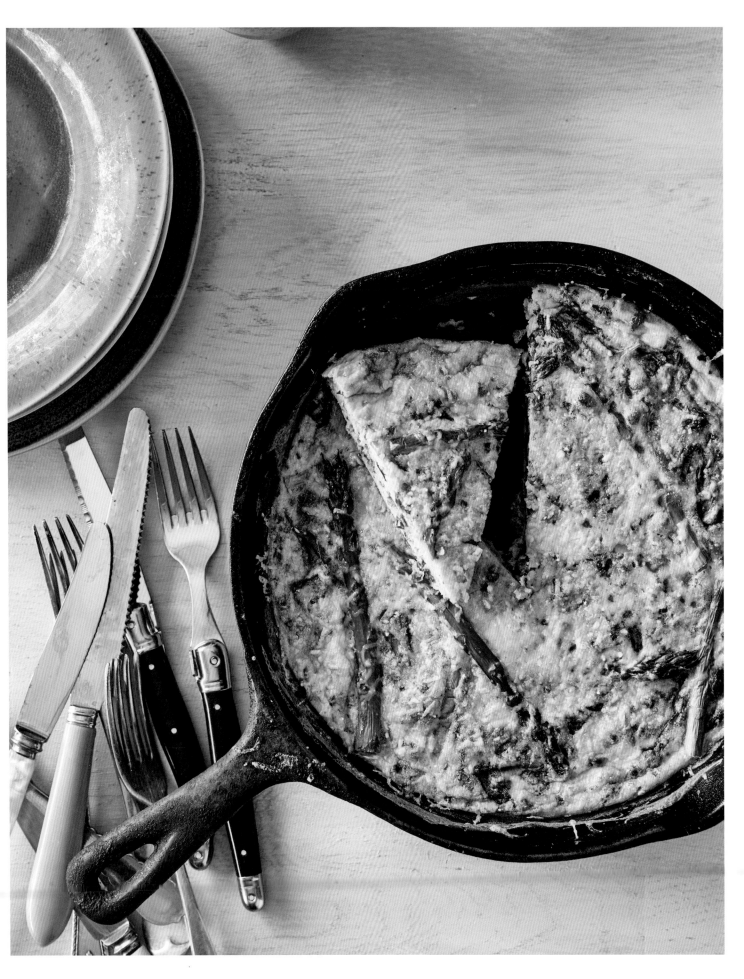

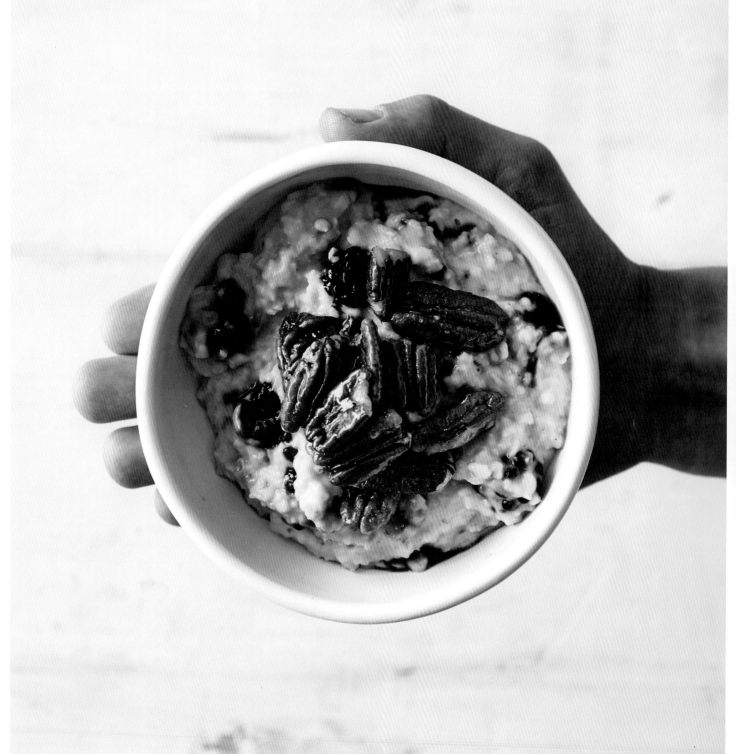

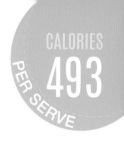

'Pimped Up' Porridge with Maple Pecans and Mixed Berries

(SERVES 1)

Porridge is the real deal when it comes to long-lasting energy.
Throw in some sweet toasted pecans and forest fruits and you are onto an epic breakfast
combo to fuel the day ahead.

You will need:

½ cup 'quick' oats

½ handful raw pecans

½ cup frozen mixed berries

1 tbs maple syrup

½ handful sunflower seeds

1 ½ cups almond milk

pinch of salt

Simple steps:

Preheat the oven to 180°C (350°F). Line a small oven tray with baking paper. Scatter the pecans on the tray and add a pinch of salt. Roast in the oven for 15 minutes. About 5 minutes before the nuts are ready, remove from the oven and drizzle with maple syrup, then return to the oven for the remaining time.

Put the oats, sunflower seeds, and almond milk in a pan and heat gently over a medium heat. Cook for 3–4 minutes, stirring regularly. Add a dash of water or extra almond milk if the porridge needs it then stir in the mixed berries and remove from the heat. Top with the maple pecans. Be careful as the maple syrup will still be very hot.

TOP TIP:

Roast some extra pecans, then once cool, store in an airtight container ready for the next bowl of delicious porridge. They are also great to nibble on when you're peckish.

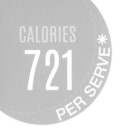

Cheat's Huevos Rancheros

(SERVES 2)

I have been known to eat this super-hearty Mexican breakfast for lunch ... OK,
and for dinner. But don't judge me. Once you've made it, you'll understand.

You will need:

2 wholemeal tortillas

2 tomatoes, roughly chopped

1 red onion, finely diced

1 garlic clove, finely diced

1 lime, zested and juiced

½ tin, 220 g (7 oz), refried beans

3 tbs cottage cheese

4 eggs

1 red chilli, finely sliced

½ avocado, sliced

1 bunch coriander (cilantro), roughly chopped

1–2 tsp green chilli sauce (habanero)

2 tbs extra virgin olive oil

salt and pepper

Simple steps:

Preheat the oven to full power, or if you have a pizza oven turn it up to full power.

Heat a dry pan over a medium heat and cook the tortillas for 2–3 minutes on each side, until they start to color. Remove and place on a large chopping board.

Put the tomato, red onion and garlic in a small bowl and season with salt, pepper and a drizzle of olive oil. Add the lime zest and half the juice to the bowl and mix well.

Spread the refried beans evenly over the tortilla and top with a generous serving of tomato salsa and cottage cheese.

Gently fry two eggs at a time in a pan with a little olive oil. Remove the eggs from the pan just before they are cooked. The yolk should be very runny but still holding its shape. Place two eggs onto one tortilla then scatter with cheese and fresh chillies.

If you are using an oven, place the tortillas onto a large tray and bake together, otherwise cook individually in the pizza oven. The regular oven will take about 5–6 minutes while the pizza oven only 2–3 minutes.

Once cooked top with avocado and coriander, finishing with chilli sauce and fresh lime juice.

TOP TIP:

Refried beans make for a great dip. Simply slice some cucumber, carrot and celery into sticks and dip in.

* Need this recipe a little lighter?
Simply reduce the olive oil 1 tbs (20ml) olive oil = 165 calories

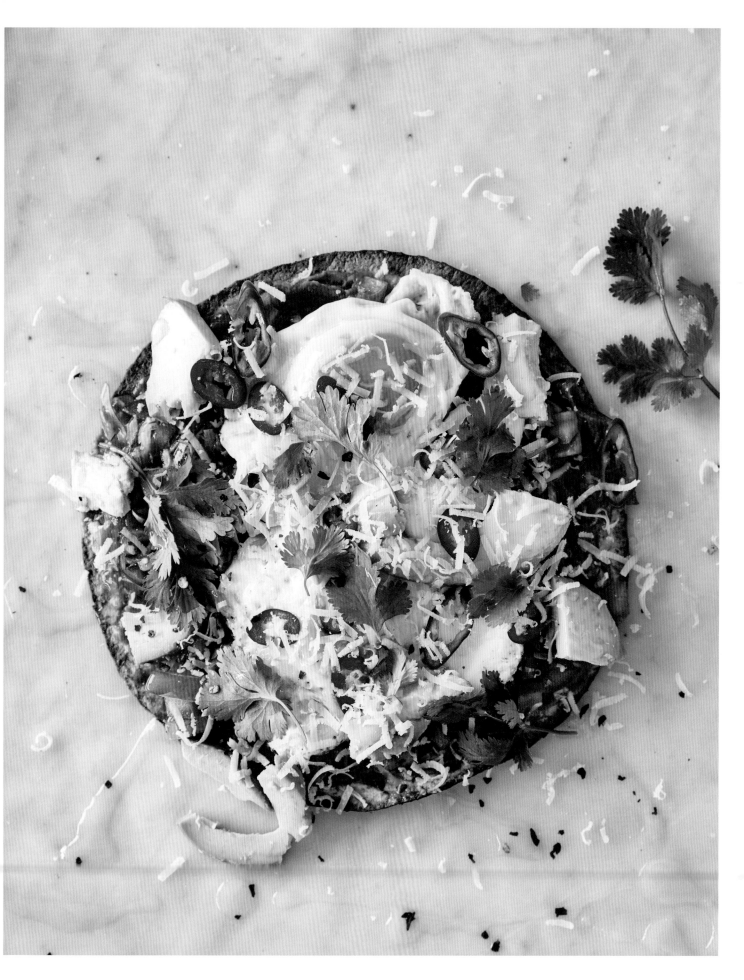

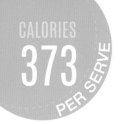

CALORIES

373

PER SERVE

Morning Grapefruit and Granola

(SERVES 1)

Ahh the good old grapefruit! Segmented and served with crunchy granola
it's a match made in breakfast heaven.

You will need:

½ cup 'Too Good' toasted granola
(see page 41)

1 grapefruit

2 tbs full fat natural yoghurt

100 ml (3 fl oz) milk of your choice

Simple steps:

Spoon the 'Too Good' toasted granola into a breakfast bowl. Segment the grapefruit, then squeeze the remaining grapefruit over the top of the granola. Add the yoghurt to the granola and finish with grapefruit segments, and if you fancy it add a dash of your choice of milk.

GOOD TO KNOW:

Grapefruit is jam-packed with **vitamin C**, which acts as an antioxidant for our body. Good times!

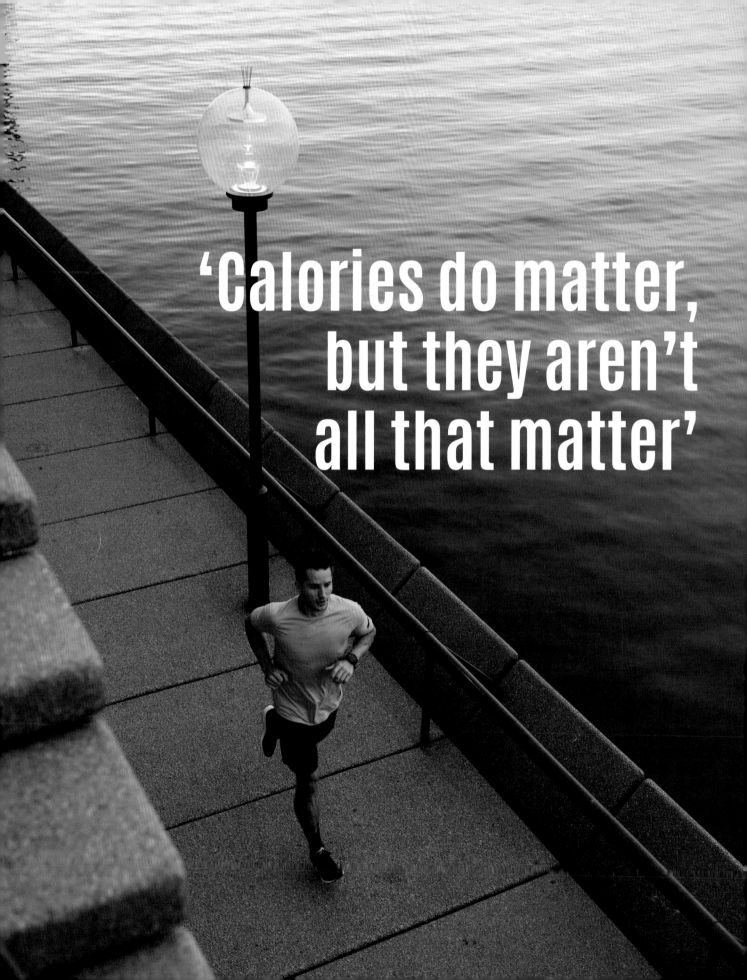

'Calories do matter,
but they aren't
all that matter'

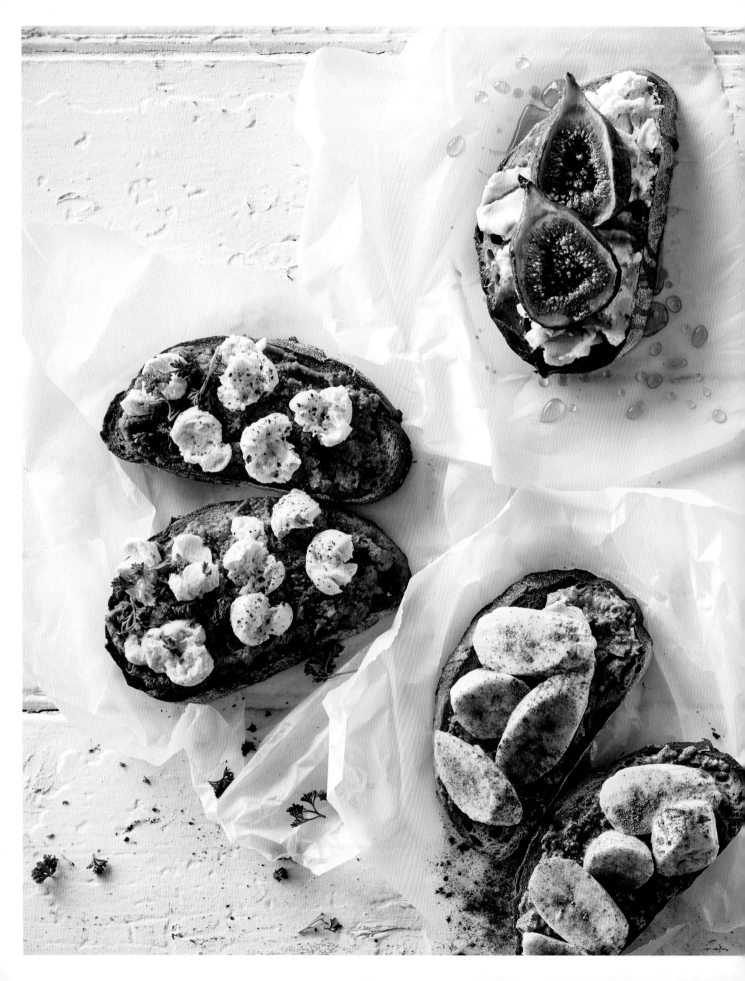

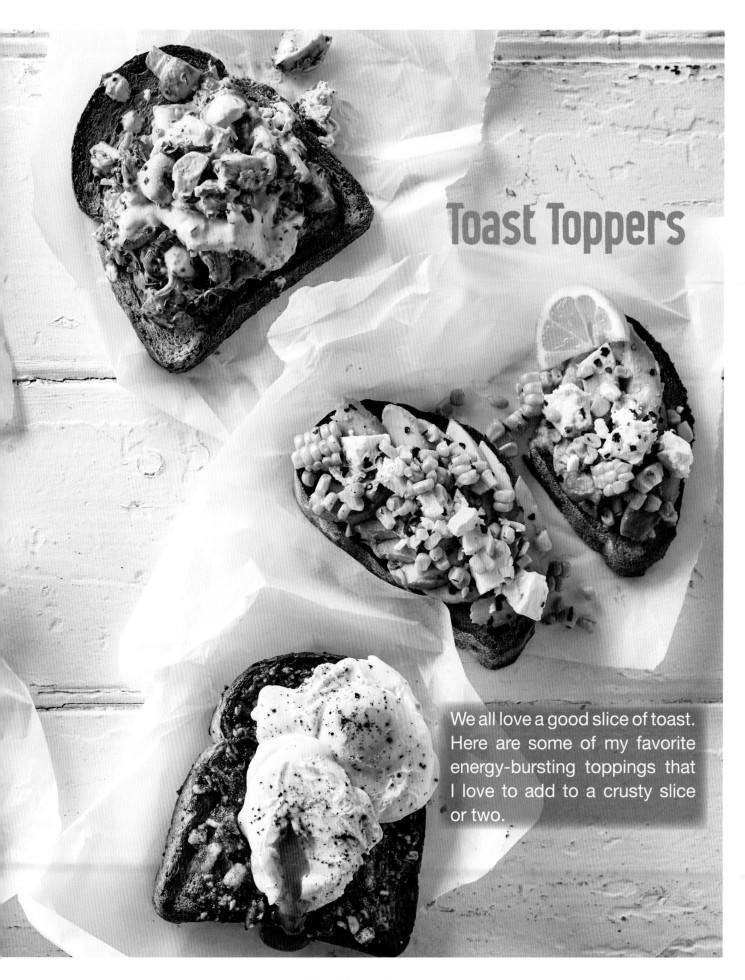

Toast Toppers

We all love a good slice of toast. Here are some of my favorite energy-bursting toppings that I love to add to a crusty slice or two.

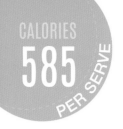

Avo, Feta and Roasted Chilli Corn

(EACH RECIPE SERVES 1)

Spicy, salty and sweet this is a cracking combo.

You will need:

- 1 corn cob
- ½ tsp dried chilli flakes
- 2 small slices wholemeal bread
- ¼ avocado, sliced
- 25 g (0.8 oz) feta cheese, crumbled
- ¼ lemon, juiced
- 1 tbs extra virgin olive oil
- salt and pepper

Simple steps:

Preheat the grill to its maximum temperature setting. Place the corn on an oven tray, drizzle a little olive oil and sprinkle with chilli flakes and a little salt. Rub the seasoning all over the corn then grill for 5 minutes. Roll the corn over and grill for another 5 minutes.

Toast the bread then once cooked lay the avocado on each slice and top with crumbled feta, chilli flakes and a drizzle of olive oil. Season with pepper only. Stand the corn on its end and carefully slice the corn off the cob using a sharp knife. Sprinkle over the top of the toast. Finish with a squeeze of fresh lemon juice.

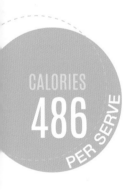

Peanut Butter, Banana and Cinnamon

The perfect energy boost before a long run.

You will need:

- 2 small slices sourdough bread
- 2 tbs peanut butter, chunky or smooth
- 1 medium banana sliced
- ½ tsp ground cinnamon

Simple steps:

Toast the bread then spread the peanut butter on the toast. Add the sliced banana and top with a light sprinkling of cinnamon powder.

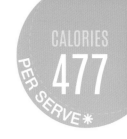

Grilled Goat's Cheese and Glazed Figs

Just the topping when you're looking for a little indulgence.

You will need:

- 2 figs, halved
- 1 tsp honey
- 2 small slices sourdough bread
- 25 g (0.8 oz) soft goat's cheese
- 1 tbs extra virgin olive oil

Simple steps:

Preheat the oven to 180°C (350°F). Putl Place the figs onto an oven tray and drizzle honey over the top. Roast in the oven for 10 minutes until soft.

Toast the bread then lay the figs on top. Crumble the feta cheese over the top of the figs then drizzle with a little olive oil and grill for 60 seconds, keeping an eye on the toast to ensure it doesn't burn. Top with a little extra honey if you like and serve.

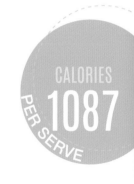

Chunky Almond Pesto and Soft Poached Egg

Just the protein hit you're looking for first thing in the morning

You will need:

- ½ bunch fresh basil
- ½ handful almonds
- 1 garlic clove, crushed
- 25 g (0.8 oz) parmesan cheese
- 4 tbs extra virgin olive oil
- 2 eggs, poached
- white wine vinegar
- 1 large slice of wholemeal bread
- salt and pepper

Simple steps:

To make the pesto, put the basil leaves, almonds, garlic, parmesan cheese and olive oil in a blender and blend. I like to keep mine fairly chunky but if you like it smooth just keep blending. Season well with salt and pepper and give it one final quick pulse.

Heat a pan of water on the stove to a simmer, so you can see small rolling bubbles. Add a dash of white wine vinegar then crack an egg into a small cup and carefully tip the egg into the simmering water. Repeat with another egg then allow them to cook gently for 2–3 minutes.

Once cooked use a slotted spoon and carefully lift the eggs out of the water and onto a tea towel or a piece of kitchen paper to drain the excess water.

Toast the bread then spread with pesto. Top with a poached egg and season with some cracked black pepper and a drizzle of olive oil.

* Need this recipe a little lighter?
Simply reduce the olive oil 1 tbs (20ml) olive oil = 165 calories

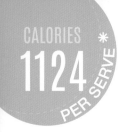

Sun-Dried Tomato Hummus with Bocconcini

Delicious, but extremely addictive, it may never actually make it onto the toast …

You will need:

2 small slices sourdough bread

tin (100g/3.5 oz) garbanzo beans

6 sun-dried tomatoes

½ tbs tahini

4 tbs extra virgin olive oil

½ a lemon, zested and juiced

¼ bunch parsley, chopped

25 g (1.7 oz) bocconcini cheese

salt and pepper

Simple steps:

Rinse and drain the chickpeas. Place in a blender along with the sun-dried tomatoes, tahini, olive oil, lemon zest and juice, and season with salt and pepper. Blend until the chickpeas come together.

Add the fresh parsley and give it one final pulse. I like to keep my hummus fairly chunky but if you like it smooth keep on blending.

Toast the bread then spread generously with the hummus. Tear the bocconcini into small pieces and arrange over the top. Finish with some fresh lemon juice and extra pepper.

TOP TIP:

Double up on the hummus, store in the refrigerator then serve up with some vegetable sticks, crackers or bread sticks for a super-easy snack.

* Need this recipe a little lighter?
Simply reduce the olive oil 1 tbs (20ml) olive oil = 165 calories

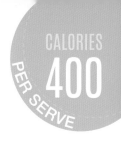

Cheesy Chive Mushrooms

Creamy cheesy mushrooms ... enough said

You will need:

¼ onion, finely diced

½ a garlic clove, finely diced

8–10 button mushrooms, quartered

2 heaped tbs sour cream

1 handful spinach

25 g (0.8 oz) parmesan cheese

1 small slice wholemeal bread

¼ bunch chives, finely chopped

2 tbs extra virgin olive oil

salt and pepper

Simple steps:

Pan fry the onion, garlic and mushrooms in a pan with a little olive oil over a medium heat for 3–4 minutes. Season well with salt and pepper. Spoon in the sour cream and stir. Add the spinach and allow to soften then add the parmesan cheese and remove the pan from the heat. Toast the bread and serve the mushrooms on the toast topped with chopped chives.

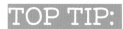

TOP TIP:

Double up on the portions, store in the refrigerator then serve up with some rice for a super-quick lunch or dinner. Tastes delicious with a piece of chicken or salmon.

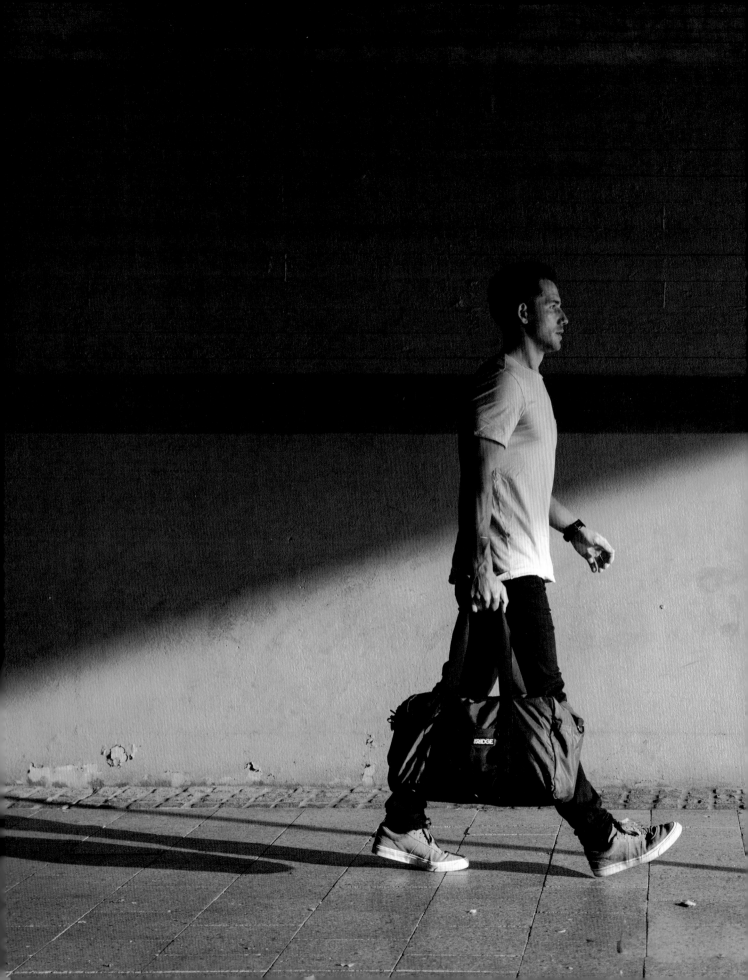

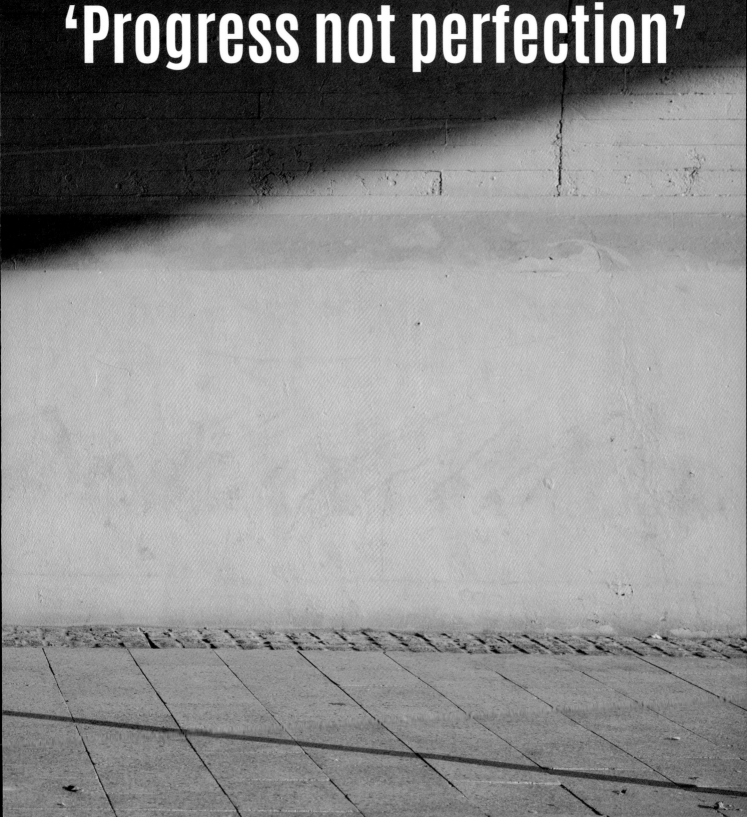

'Progress not perfection'

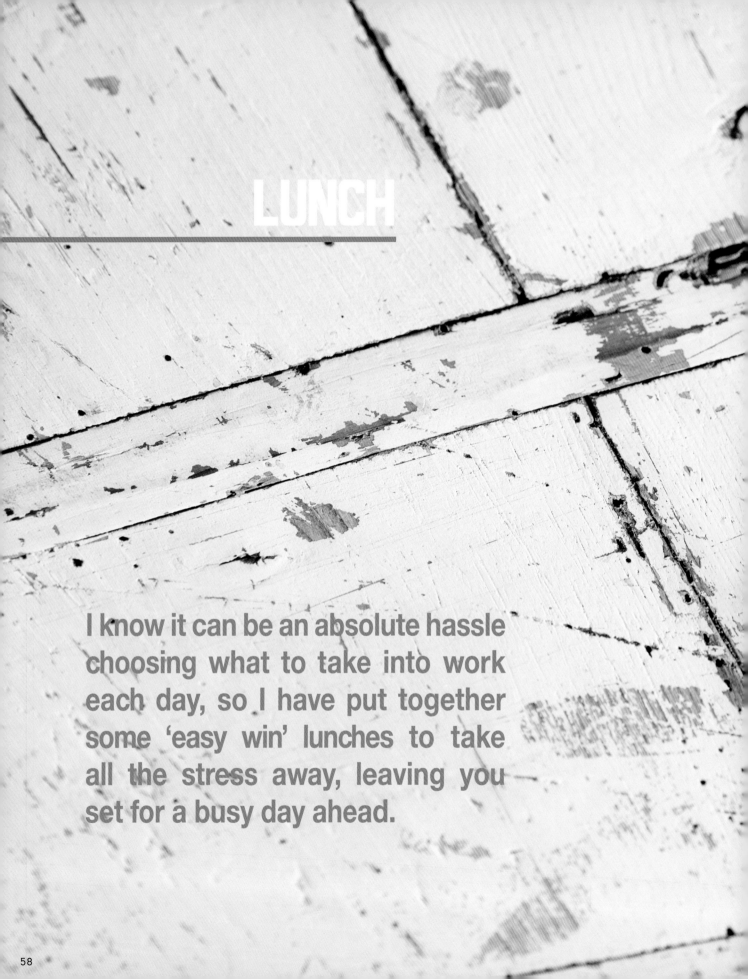

LUNCH

I know it can be an absolute hassle choosing what to take into work each day, so I have put together some 'easy win' lunches to take all the stress away, leaving you set for a busy day ahead.

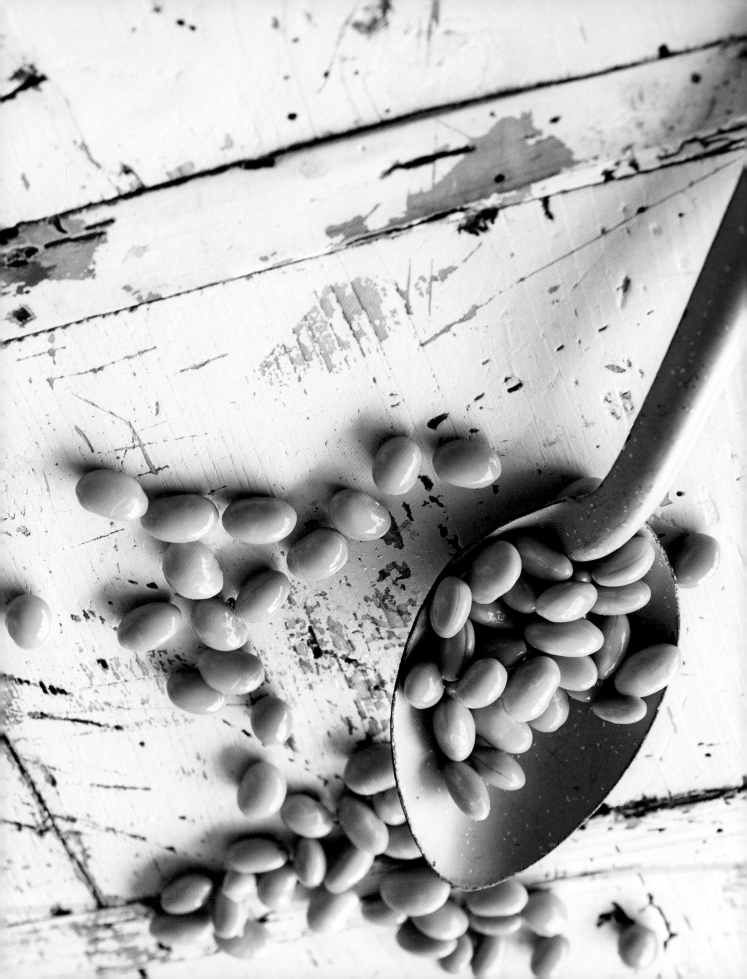

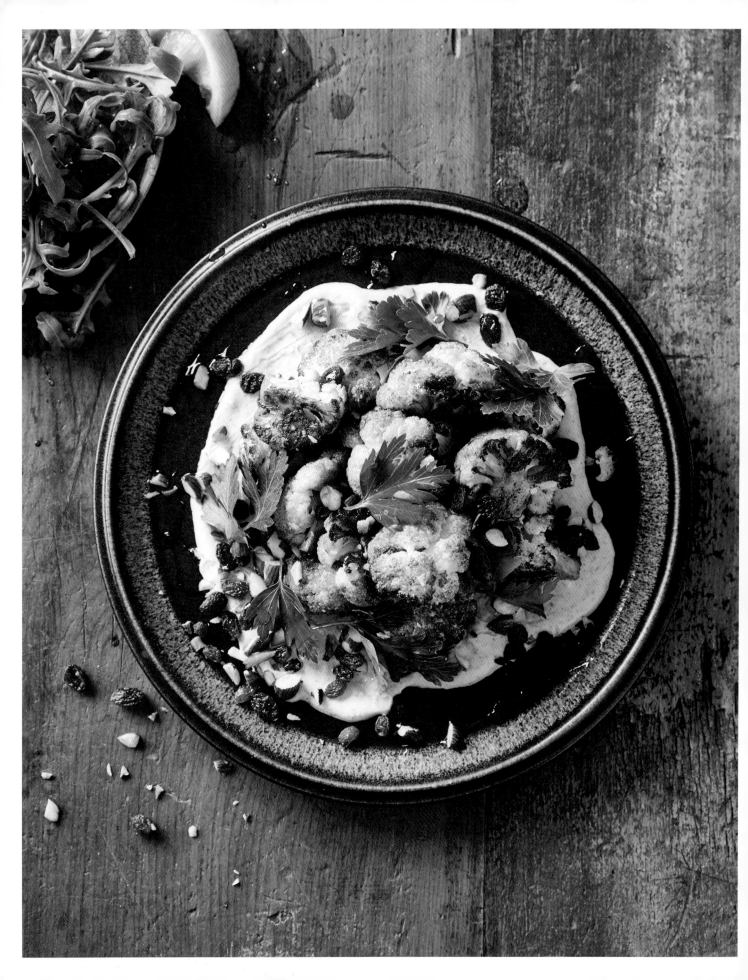

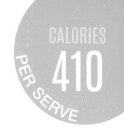

Turmeric Roasted Cauliflower with Minted Yoghurt

(SERVES 2)

Turmeric not only adds a vibrant color but also a wonderfully nutty flavor to cauliflower, plus roasting the cauliflower in the oven creates caramelized edges, bringing bags of toasted yumminess.

You will need:

- 1 medium-sized cauliflower, cut into florets
- 2 tsp ground turmeric
- 1 handful roasted almonds, roughly chopped
- ½ bunch fresh parsley
- 1 handful sultanas, roughly chopped
- 3–4 tbs yoghurt
- 1 bunch fresh mint, very finely chopped
- 1 lemon, zested
- 1 tbs honey
- 1 bag rocket (arugula)
- 1 tbs extra virgin olive oil
- salt and pepper

Simple steps

Preheat the oven to 200°C (390°F). Place the cauliflower in a large bowl with the turmeric, a good drizzle of olive oil and a generous twist of salt and pepper. Rub the spice and seasoning into the cauliflower with your hands, ensuring it's evenly covered. Transfer the cauliflower to an oven tray and roast for 16–18 minutes. Allow the corners of the cauliflower to start to burn a little as this adds a lovely toasted flavor. Five minutes before removing the cauliflower throw in the almonds and sultanas and give the tray a good shake, then return the tray to the oven to finish cooking. Once the cauliflower is cooked add some fresh parsley and mix well.

To make the minted yoghurt, put spoon the yoghurt in into a bowl and stir in the very finely chopped mint, lemon zest, honey and a good pinch of salt and pepper. (The finer you can chop the mint the greener the yoghurt will be.)

Spread the yoghurt on a plate then top with the cauliflower florets, almonds and sultanas. Serve with a side of rocket salad and a squeeze of fresh lemon juice.

GOOD TO KNOW:

Turmeric is actually a member of the ginger family and is thought to have superb **healing properties**.

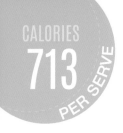

Halloumi and Watermelon Summer Salad

(SERVES 2)

Perfect for a light lunch or as part of a main meal, pan-fried halloumi is the rock star of the cheese world. Throw it together with chunks of juicy watermelon and you've got a salad that's worth shouting about.

You will need:

180 g (6.5 oz) halloumi, sliced 1 cm (0.3 in) thick

1 lemon

10 cherry tomatoes, sliced in half

¼ red onion, very finely sliced

4 radishes, finely sliced

½ avocado, diced

½ a cucumber, peeled into strips

2 baby gem lettuce, shredded

2 large slices watermelon, cut into chunks

Honey mustard dressing:

2 tbs extra virgin olive oil

2 tbs white wine vinegar

1 tsp honey

1 tsp Dijon mustard

pinch salt and pepper

Simple steps:

Pan fry the halloumi in a dry non-stick pan over a medium heat. After about 60 seconds turn each piece over and fry for another 60 seconds then squeeze lemon juice over the top and a twist of black pepper and remove from the pan.

Add the tomatoes, red onion, radish, avocado and cucumber to a bowl and mix together with your hands. Arrange the baby gem lettuce leaves around the bottom of a separate shallow dish then add the salad mix over the top of the baby gem lettuce.

To make the dressing, put all the ingredients in a jar, screw the lid on tight and give it good shake.

Slice the halloumi into strips then scatter over the top of the salad along with the chunks of watermelon. Finish by drizzling honey mustard dressing over the top and serve.

TOP TIP:

Leave the dressing separate until you are actually planning on eating the salad as it will stay nice and crunchy and super fresh.

GOOD TO KNOW:

Watermelon is **low in calories** so it's a great choice when you're looking for a light snack.

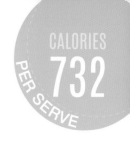

Vietnamese Rice Paper Rolls

(SERVES 2)

Rice paper rolls are the ultimate speedy snack you can eat with your hands. In my opinion, if you like the ingredients then they'll work rolled up in a rice paper roll.

You will need:

- 6 rice paper sheets
- 2 tbs chilli dipping sauce
- 250 g (8.8 oz) microwave brown rice or quinoa

Optional fillings – each makes 2 rolls:

- 200 g (7 oz) sliced chicken/4 tbs cottage cheese/8–10 basil leaves/1 carrot very finely sliced
- 90 g (3 oz) smoked salmon /1 tsp wasabi paste /2 handfuls cress/½ capsicum thinly sliced
- 90 g tuna (3 oz) /1 tbs mayonnaise / 2 handfuls spinach / ½ cucumber thinly sliced

Simple steps:

Prepare one sheet of rice paper at a time. Dip the rice paper into a shallow dish of warm water for 8–10 seconds and allow to soften. Place a large damp cloth on a chopping board then carefully lay the rice paper on top. Put a little bit of rice in the middle of the paper then top with your chosen filling in any order you like. Fold the bottom of the paper up to meet the filling then pull each side over the top, securing the filling in tightly.

Transfer to a clean plate and place a damp cloth on top then start with the next roll (this will stop the rolls from drying out). Once complete place the rolls in a container, cover and store in the fridge.

Serve with chilli dipping sauce.

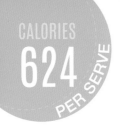

Spicy Prawn Wraps with Whipped Avo and Mango Salsa

(SERVES 1)

Succulent juicy prawns topped with creamy avocado and packed into a soft tortilla is my kind of fast food.

You will need:

½ avocado, diced

1 tsp tahini

1 garlic clove, crushed

¼ tsp chilli flakes

1 lemon, zested and juiced

1 medium wholemeal wrap

2 large handfuls rocket (arugula) leaves

½ medium-sized red capsicum (bell pepper), finely sliced

130 g (4.5 oz) cooked prawns

½ a mango, diced

salt and pepper

Simple steps:

Put the avocado, tahini, garlic, chilli flakes, lemon zest and a pinch of salt and pepper into a small mixing bowl. Use a stick blender and pulse until smooth.

Spread the avocado generously in the middle of each wrap. Add a small handful of rocket, capsicum and cooked prawns. Top with diced mango and a squeeze of lemon juice. Fold the end of the wrap up to meet the filling in the middle then bring one side of the wrap over the top and roll, tightly, securing all of the filling.

TOP TIP:

The unfilled wraps freeze really well. Simply defrost in the microwave for 30–45 seconds right before you want to use them then ensure you wrap them tightly with cling film to stop them from drying out.

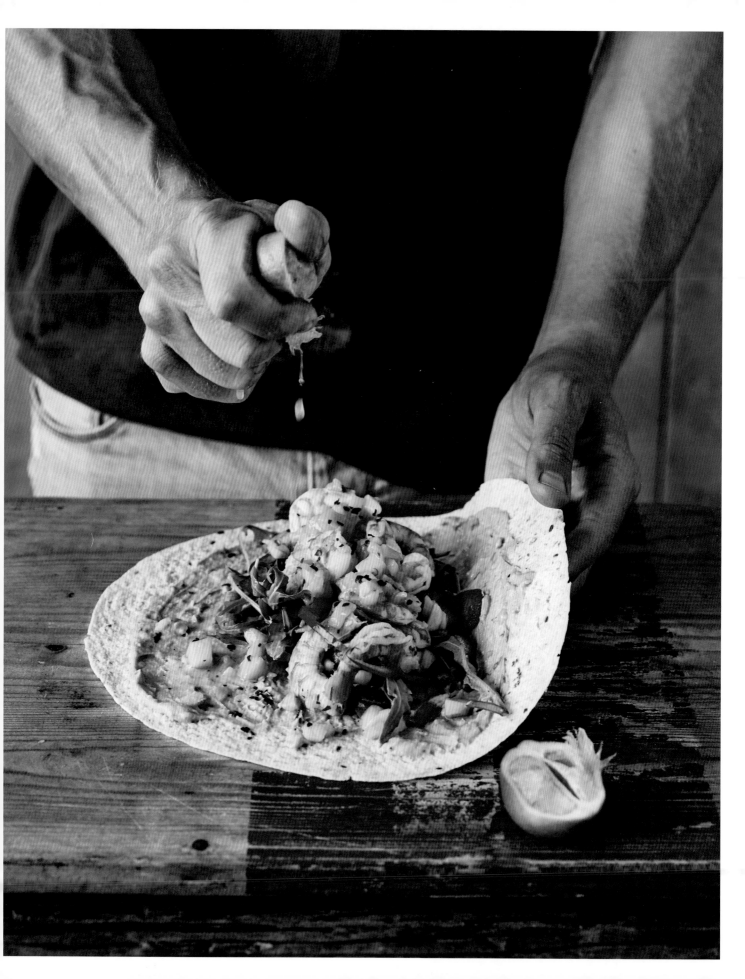

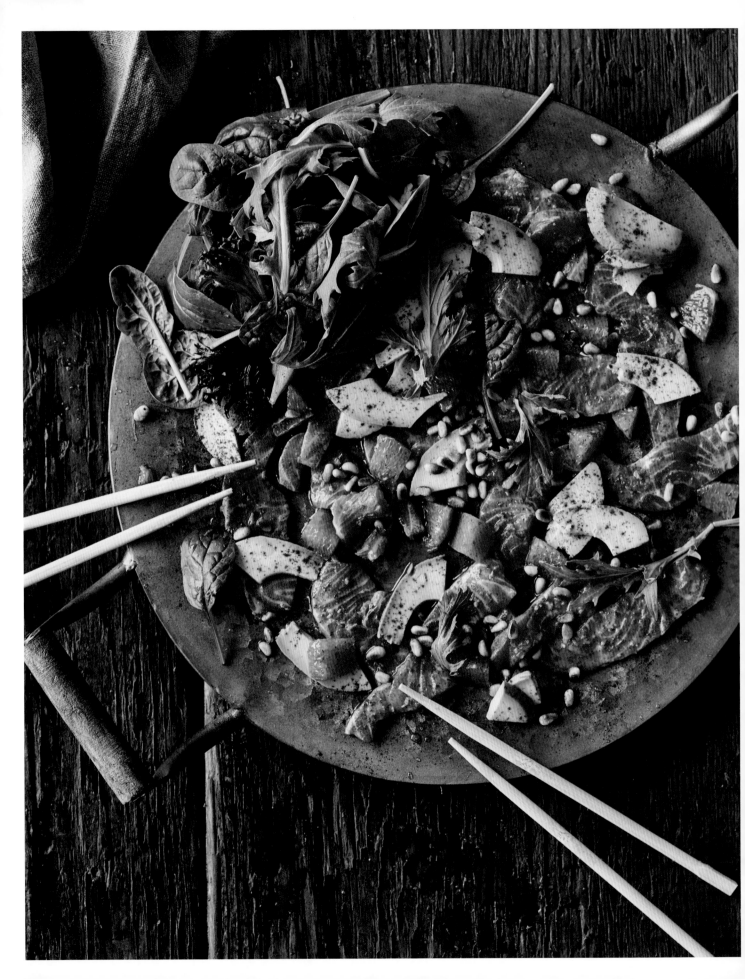

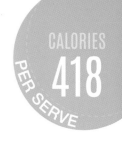

Salmon Ceviche with Grapefruit and Lime

(SERVES 2)

Fresh, zingy and packed full of good fats, salmon ceviche is delicious and I'm seriously obsessed with it! The citrus gently cooks the fish making it unbelievably tender and moreish.

You will need:

2 skinless salmon fillets (super fresh)

1 grapefruit, segmented

1 lime, zested and juiced

1 tsp honey

2 tbs pine nuts, toasted

½ avocado, sliced

1 small bag mixed salad leaves

1 tsp paprika

salt and pepper

Simple steps:

Slice the salmon into very thin slices and lay on a plate or shallow dish.

Slice the grapefruit into segments then roughly chop into small pieces. In a small bowl combine the zest and juice of the lime, the grapefruit segments and honey, and season with salt and pepper. Squeeze the remaining grapefruit into the bowl to extract as much juice as possible. Stir well then place a few spoons of the mix over the salmon and leave for 2–3 minutes. Leave a little dressing to one side for the mixed leaves.

While the dressing is doing its thing, toast the pine nuts in a dry pan over a medium heat for 2–3 minutes until golden brown.

Add the sliced avocado to the mixed leaves and top with a little extra dressing.

Place the salmon onto a large serving plate, sprinkle with a little paprika, and serve with the salad. Sprinkle the toasted pine nuts over the salmon along with any leftover dressing. Finally add a generous twist of salt and pepper and a drizzle of olive oil.

TOP TIP:

Whenever you eat fish ensure it's **super fresh**, but it's especially important when making ceviche. The citrus dressing will start to cook the salmon straight away, so if you aren't planning on eating it straight away then leave the dressing to one side and pour over when ready.

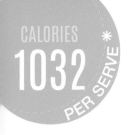

Epic Lunch Box Hummus Wraps

(SERVES 2)

Whipped up in under two minutes, hummus has to be one of the easiest dips out there.
I'm baffled as to why so many people buy it; you can always tell when a hummus
has been made from scratch. I love the nuttiness that you get from the tahini and the big,
bold flavors you can add to the chickpeas to step it up a level.

You will need:

²⁄ tin (160 g / 6 oz) garbanzo beans drained

1 garlic clove, crushed

1 lemon, juiced

1 tbs tahini

2 large wholemeal wraps

¼ cucumber, finely sliced

6–8 sliced cherry tomatoes

¼ bunch coriander (cilantro) leaves picked

¼ red cabbage, finely sliced

2 tbs natural yoghurt

extra virgin olive oil

salt and pepper

Simple steps:

Drain and rinse the chickpeas under cold water. Put in the food processor along with the garlic, half the lemon juice, tahini and about 6–8 tablespoons of olive oil (trust me, the shop-bought stuff contains a lot more!). Season well with salt and pepper.

Spread the hummus generously in the middle of the wrap. Top with the cucumber, cherry tomatoes and coriander leaves. Mix the yoghurt with a little extra the lemon juice in a small bowl then spoon over the salad. Fold the end of the wrap up to meet the filling in the middle, then bring one side of the wrap over the top and roll, securing all the filling tightly.

TOP TIP:

Double up on the recipe and store a bowl of hummus in the fridge. It's such a great snack to always have on hand that only needs a few veggie sticks or crackers as an accompaniment.

*Need this recipe a little lighter?
Simply reduce the olive oil 1 tbs (20ml) olive oil = 165 calories

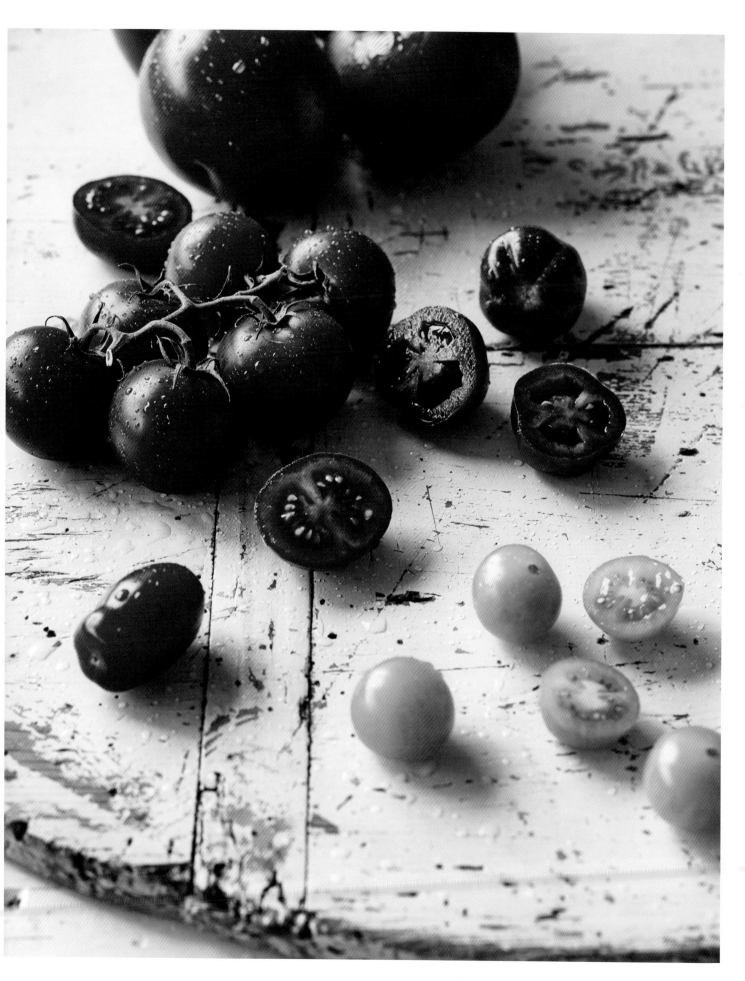

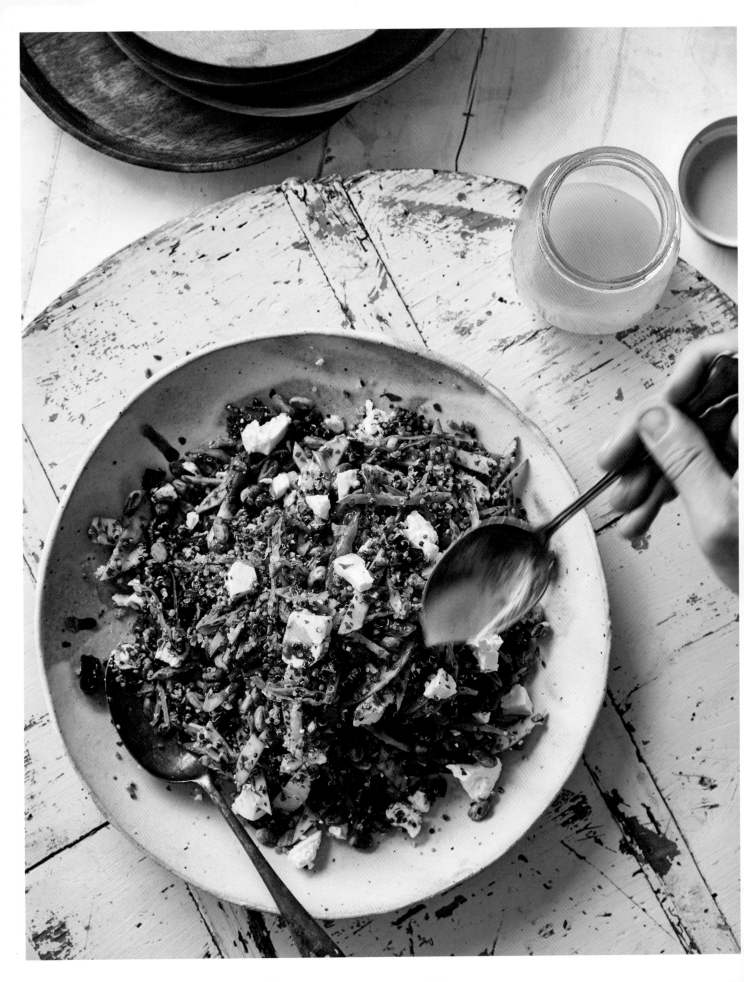

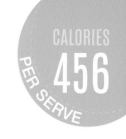

Beetroot Apple and Sugar Snap Pea Tabbouleh

(SERVES 4)

OK, so this sounds fancy, but tabbouleh is actually incredibly easy to throw together. I love making a big bowl of tabbouleh and just storing it in the fridge. It really is so good on its own, or enjoyed with some chicken or pork for that extra hit of protein.

You will need:

1 cup raw quinoa

2 bunches parsley, very finely chopped

1 apple, finely sliced into matchsticks

1 bag sugar snap peas, finely sliced

2 handfuls pistachios or almonds

2 cooked beetroot, diced into very small pieces

100 g feta cheese crumbled

salt and pepper

Honey beetroot dressing:

1 cooked beetroot, very finely chopped

1 lemon, juiced

1 tbs honey

4 tbs olive oil

2 tbs apple cider vinegar

1 garlic clove, finely grated or chopped

Simple steps:

Place the quinoa in a sieve and rinse under cold water for 30 seconds. Transfer to a saucepan along with 2 cups of water. Bring the water to the boil and stir once, then reduce the heat to a simmer. Cook for 15 minutes then remove from the heat. Rinse the quinoa under cold water to stop the cooking process then drain well one final time.

Once drained tip the quinoa into a large oval dish or plate then add the chopped parsley, apple and sugar snap peas.

To make the dressing, chop the beetroot as fine as you can, so it almost becomes like a paste, then put all the ingredients in a clean jar along with the rest of the dressing ingredients. Screw the lid on and give it a good shake.

Toast the pistachios in a dry pan over a medium heat for 2–3 minutes, shaking the pan every 30 seconds or so until golden.

Add the beetroot to the salad then drizzle with the dressing and give it a good toss. Top with crumbled feta and toasted pistachios.

TOP TIP:

If you aren't planning on eating the salad straight away, leave the dressing in the jar and store in a cool dry place. Squeeze a little extra lemon juice over the apple to prevent it from turning brown in the fridge.

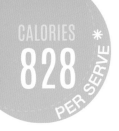

Sicilian Chilli Tuna Linguine

(SERVES 2)

When you are on the run you need something quick and easy, and it doesn't get much quicker or easier than throwing everything into one pan. My Sicilian linguine is exactly that – easy! You honestly won't believe this is made with canned tuna either.

You will need:

200 g (7 oz) linguine

2 garlic cloves, finely sliced

½ tsp chilli flakes

½ bunch parsley, finely chopped including stalks

1 tsp capers, roughly chopped

1 lemon, zested and juiced

185 g (6.7 oz) good quality tinned tuna in oil

25 g (0.8 oz) parmesan cheese

8–10 mixed olives (optional but delicious)

3 tbs extra virgin olive oil

Simple steps:

Cook the pasta in a pan of boiling water with a good pinch of salt for 9–10 minutes.

Meanwhile, heat a non-stick pan on medium heat and drizzle in a generous amount of olive oil. Fry the garlic, chilli flakes and finely chopped parsley stalks for 60 seconds. Add the capers and lemon zest then turn the heat down.

Once the linguine is cooked, drain and add to the frying pan along with a little of the pasta water, as this helps to loosen up the pasta, then give the pan a good toss. Add the parsley and flaked tuna, then top with grated parmesan cheese, an extra drizzle of olive oil and extra chilli flakes.

TOP TIP:

Use the best quality tuna you can when making this pasta dish and look out for **responsibly sourced** fish.

* Need this recipe a little lighter?
Simply reduce the olive oil 1 tbs (20ml) olive oil = 165 calories

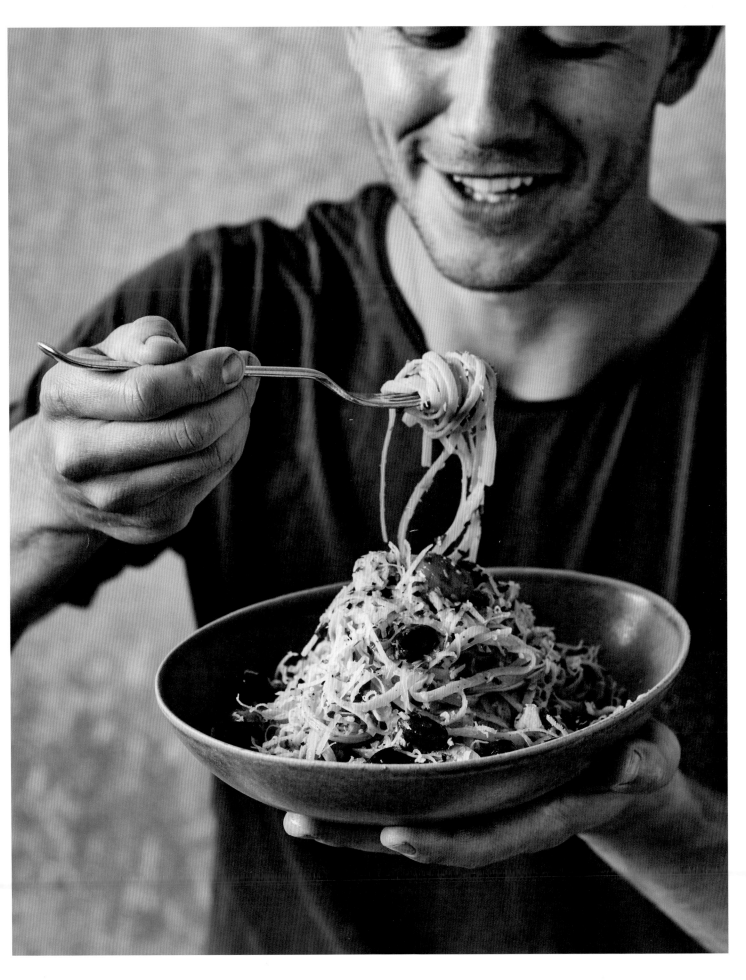

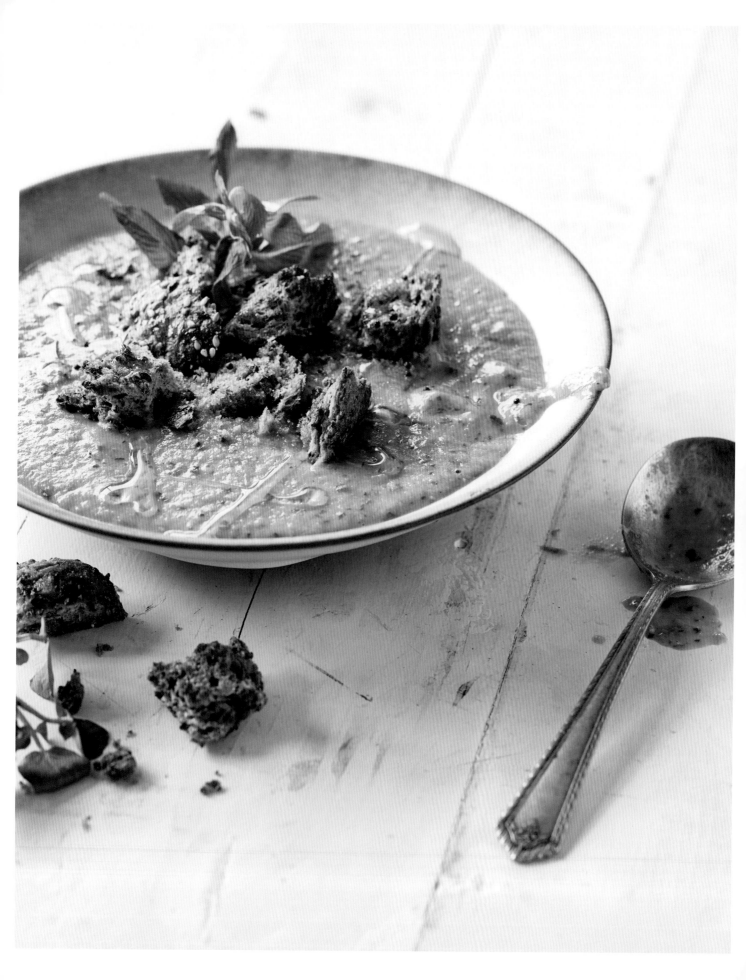

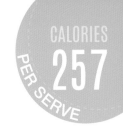

Minted Pea and Watercress Soup with Crusty Croutons

(SERVES 6)

Hearty and bursting with freshness, mint adds a wonderful kick to the soup. 'Another bowl please!'

You will need:

- 1 onion, finely diced
- 2 garlic cloves, crushed
- 2 celery stalks, finely diced
- 2 medium-sized potatoes, diced
- 1.5 litres (50 fl oz) vegetable or chicken stock
- 1 kg (2.2 lb) bag frozen peas
- 1 bunch mint, leaves picked
- 1 large bag or bunch of watercress
- 4 wholemeal rolls
- extra virgin olive oil

Simple steps:

Preheat the oven to 200°C (390°F). Fry the onion, garlic, celery and potatoes in a large pan with a little olive oil until soft. Season with a good pinch of salt and pepper.

While the veg is frying bring the stock to the boil in a separate saucepan. Add the boiling stock to the vegetables and turn the heat up so it starts to boil. Then turn the heat down slightly and cook for 5 minutes to allow the potatoes to cook. Add the peas and cook for a further 3 minutes.

Add the mint leaves to the soup along with the watercress (setting aside a few leaves to garnish later).

While the watercress and mint are softening in the soup, tear the rolls into small, bitesize pieces and scatter on an oven tray. Drizzle with olive oil and season with a little salt and pepper. Toast in the oven for 5 minutes.

Using a stick blender or food processor, blend the soup until smooth. Be very careful if you are using a food processor not to overfill the jug and ensure the lid is on tightly before blending.

Serve the soup in bowls topped with crusty croutons, a good drizzle of olive oil and the reserved watercress leaves.

TOP TIP:

Soup freezes beautifully so knock up a double or even triple batch and store in plastic containers in the freezer. Simply take out of the freezer the night before and store in the fridge ready to heat up come lunchtime.

GOOD TO KNOW:

Watercress is jam packed with **vitamin K** and extremely nutrient dense.

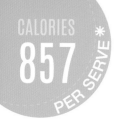

Smoked Salmon Power Bowl

(SERVES 1)

How colorful is this gorgeous bowl of goodness?! This salmon bowl has everything: nourishing healthy grains, good-for-you fats and fueling protein. The carrot and pear add some great natural sweetness to this wicked salad as well.

You will need:

½ cup frozen edamame beans

1 large carrot, grated

125 g (4.4 oz) microwave ancient grains (quinoa and brown rice)

¼ red cabbage, finely sliced

½ pear, cut into thin batons

½ yellow capsicum (bell pepper), finely sliced

90 g (3 oz) sliced smoked salmon

¼ bunch coriander (cilantro), roughly chopped

Asian dressing:

1 tbs olive oil

1 tbs sesame oil

1 tbs rice wine vinegar

1 tbs soy sauce

1 tsp honey

1 garlic clove, grated

Simple steps:

Boil the edamame beans in a pan of water for 2 minutes then rinse under cold water and drain well. Grate the carrot into a bowl then squeeze out as much of the liquid as you can with your hands; you can drink the juice, it's delicious.

To build your bowl start by microwaving the ancient grains, following the instructions on the packet, then tip into a serving bowl. Arrange the red cabbage, carrot, pear, edamame beans and capsicum around the outside of the rice, then fill the middle with slices of smoked salmon.

To make the dressing, put all of the ingredients in a clean jar, screw the lid on tightly and give it a good shake. Spoon the dressing over the top and finish with some fresh coriander leaves.

TOP TIP:

Once you have sliced all of the vegetables, you can add your favorite protein to this salad. Chicken, beef, pork and even boiled eggs all work really well.

GOOD TO KNOW:

Along with being an excellent source of protein, quinoa is also bursting with vitamins and minerals like **iron, potassium and vitamin E.**

* Need this recipe a little lighter?
Simply reduce the olive oil 1 tbs (20ml) olive oil = 165 calories

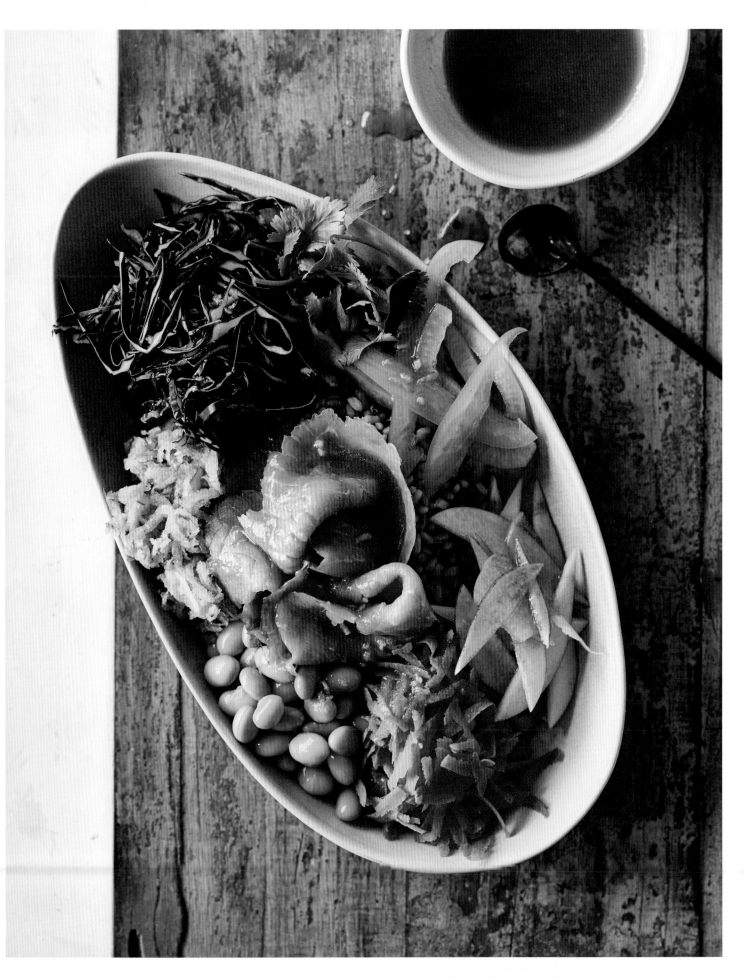

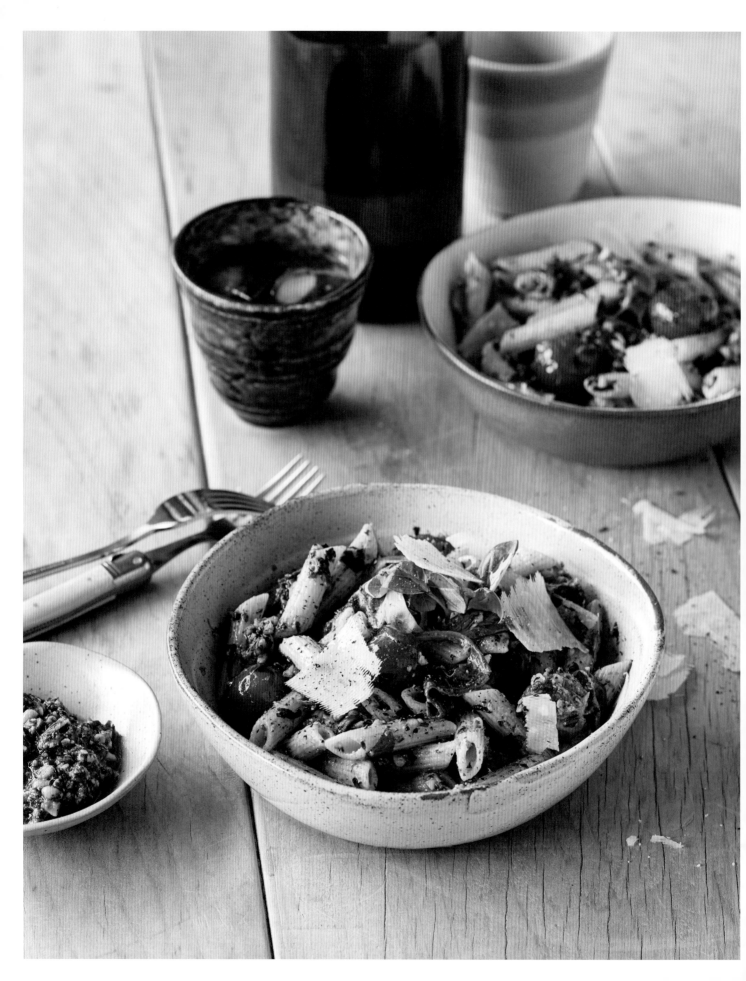

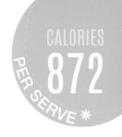

Penne Pasta with 'Kick-Ass' Pesto

(SERVES 2)

Carb me up with this banging bowl of 'kick-ass' pesto that's good enough to eat straight off the spoon. I'm confident enough to say you'll never buy it from the store again.

You will need:

- 200 g (7oz) dried penne pasta
- 1 bunch basil, leaves picked
- 4 garlic cloves, finely sliced
- ½ tsp chilli flakes
- 25 g (0.8 oz) parmesan cheese
- 1 handful pine nuts, toasted
- 80 ml extra virgin olive oil
- 12 cherry tomatoes
- 2 large handfuls spinach

Simple steps:

Cook the pasta in a pan of boiling salted water for 10–12 minutes then drain and drizzle a little olive oil over the top to stop it sticking together.

To make the pesto simply add the basil leaves, three garlic cloves, chilli flakes, parmesan cheese, pine nuts (toasted in a dry pan for 2–3 minutes) and olive oil to a food processor and give it a good pulse. Keep it fairly chunky to add some texture to the pasta. Leave a couple of basil leaves and about a tablespoon of parmesan to one side.

Heat a non-stick pan over medium heat and drizzle a little olive oil into the pan. Add the cherry tomatoes and toss regularly. After a few minutes and once they start to blister and burst, grate the final garlic clove into the pan. Reduce the heat then continue to fry for another couple of minutes then remove the pan from the heat. Add the pasta to the garlic tomatoes along with the pesto and spinach and give it a good toss. Once the spinach has softened, serve with fresh basil leaves and an extra sprinkling of parmesan cheese.

TOP TIP:

Trust me, you'll want to make some extra portions of pesto because you will be adding it to everything. Try spreading it over a roasted chicken breast and serve alongside some roasted vegetables.

GOOD TO KNOW:

Adding raw garlic into your diet can help your body's immune system, as it contains a good amount of **vitamin C.**

* Need this recipe a little lighter?
Simply reduce the olive oil 1 tbs (20ml) olive oil = 165 calories

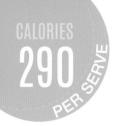

'Lean Up' Lentil and Mushroom Stir Fry (Vegan)

(SERVES 2)

Stir fries are such a great way to get a load of good nutrition into your body. Surprisingly filling for being so low in calories, this is one bowl that's just very, very tasty.

You will need:

100 g (3.5 oz) mushrooms, sliced

2 garlic cloves, finely sliced

1 fresh chilli, finely sliced

2 tbs dukkah spice mix

400 g (14 oz) tin cooked lentils

250 g (8.8 oz) sliced stir fry mix – kale, carrots, beetroot, onion

5 tbs soy sauce

½ lemon

2 tbs coconut yoghurt

extra virgin olive oil

Simple steps:

Heat a large non-stick pan over a medium heat. Drizzle a little oil in the pan and fry the mushrooms, garlic and chilli flakes. Add the dukkah spice and cook for 1–2 minutes.

Drain and rinse the lentils well under cold water. Add the stir fry mix to the pan and toss for a minute. Add the lentils along with the soy sauce and fry for another 2 minutes. Remove the pan from the heat and squeeze fresh lemon juice over the top. Serve with a spoon of coconut yoghurt.

TOP TIP:

If you're in a hurry, don't waste time chopping stir fried veg, buy it pre-sliced, ready to fry in seconds. It's 100% cheating and 100% encouraged!

GOOD TO KNOW:

This dish includes three of your five-a-day vegetables, while keeping your blood sugar levels stable.

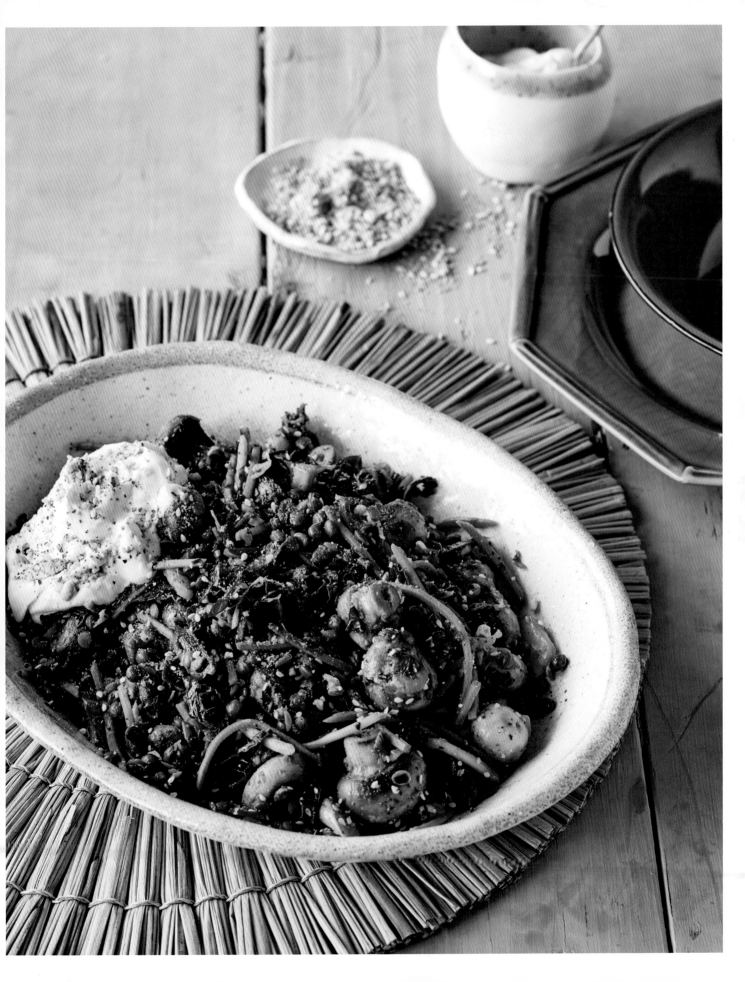

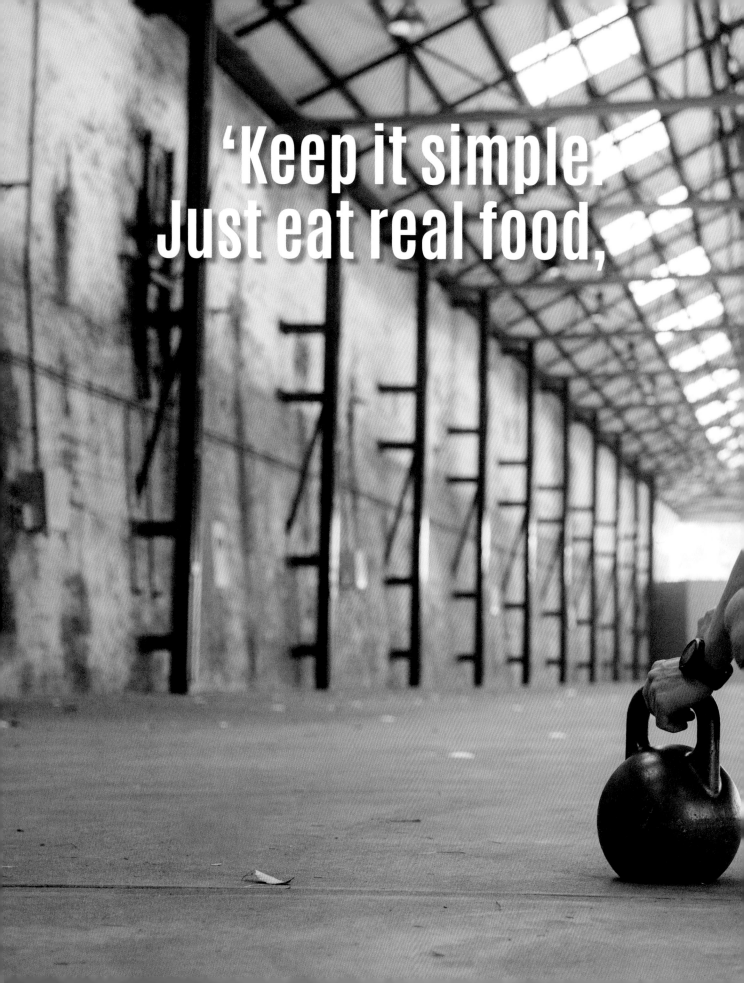

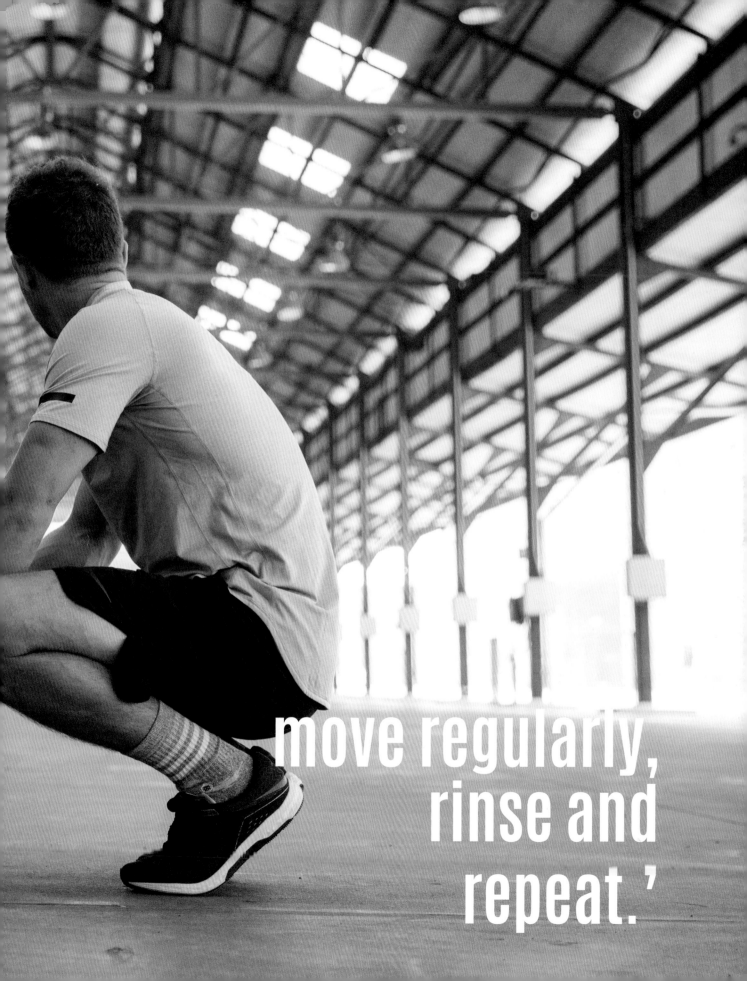

move regularly, rinse and repeat. '

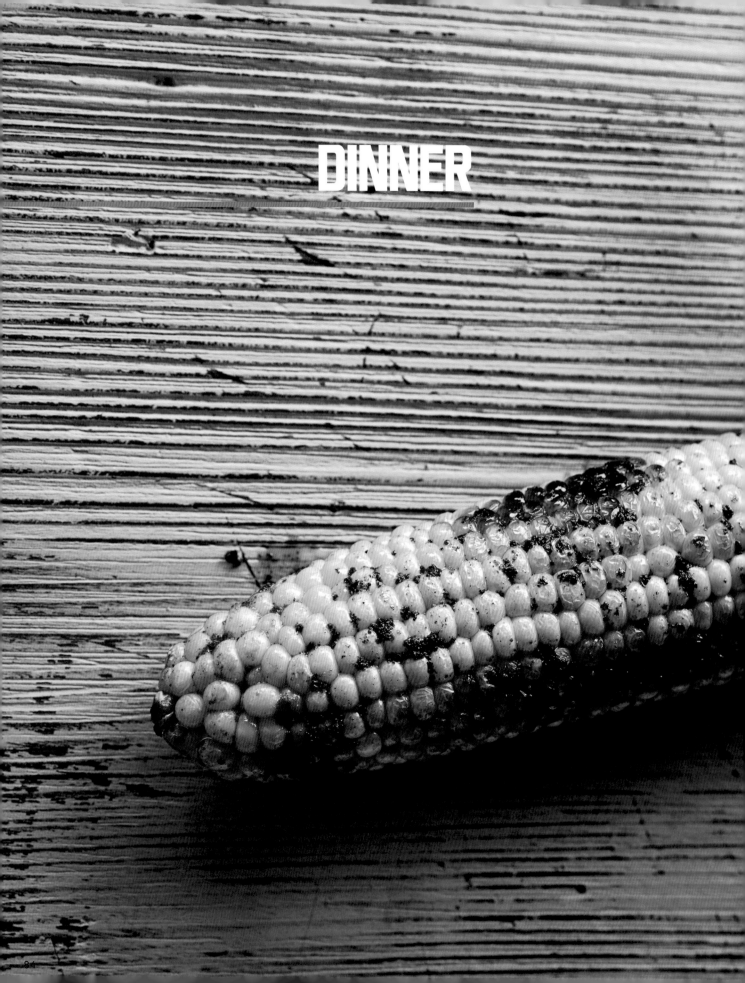

DINNER

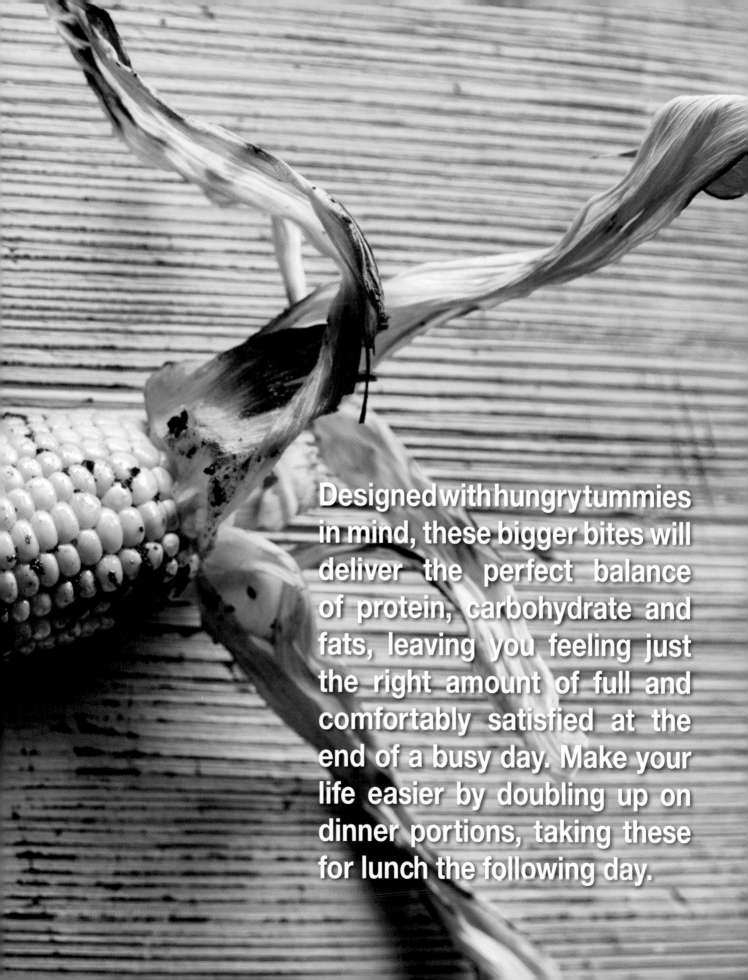

Designed with hungry tummies in mind, these bigger bites will deliver the perfect balance of protein, carbohydrate and fats, leaving you feeling just the right amount of full and comfortably satisfied at the end of a busy day. Make your life easier by doubling up on dinner portions, taking these for lunch the following day.

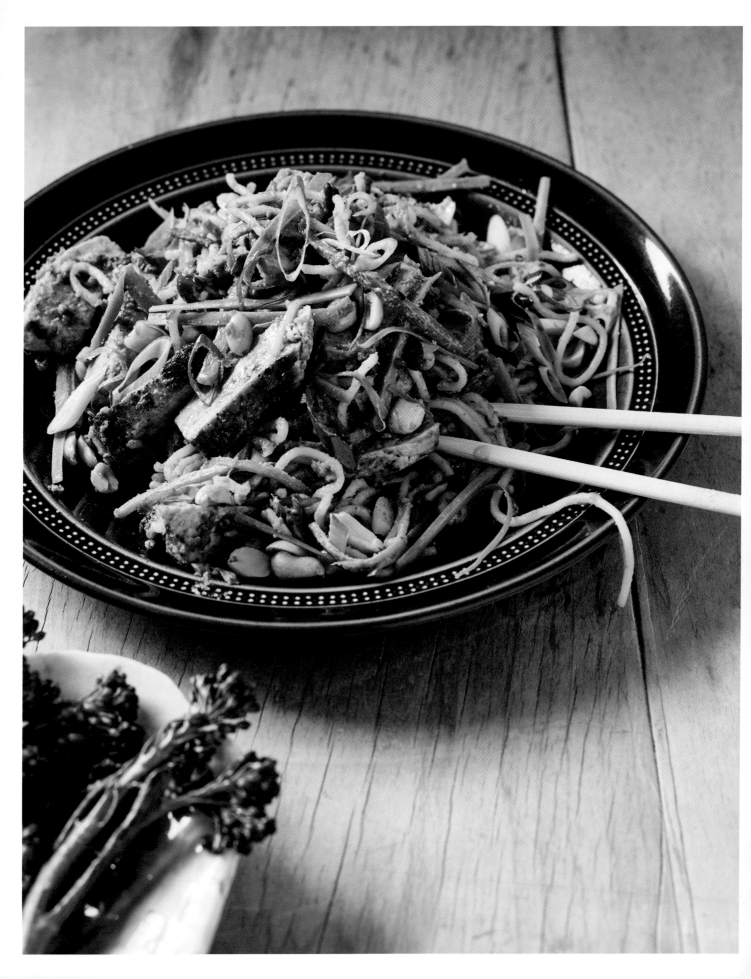

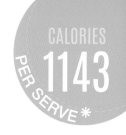

Pork with Sticky Ginger and Peanut Noodles

(SERVES 2)

I'm totally nuts about the sweet, salty and spicy flavors in this dish. The peanut sauce is such a great combo that works with just about any meat, but pork had to take the spot alongside the noodles.

You will need:

2 pork steaks

1 lime, zested and juiced

2 bunches broccolini

2 cloves garlic, finely sliced

1 carrot, finely sliced

200 g (7 oz) low-cal noodles (wok ready)

½ bunch spring onions (scallions), finely sliced

1 handful unsalted peanuts

3 tbs extra virgin olive oil

salt and pepper

Sticky ginger and peanut sauce:

3 tbs chunky peanut butter (low sugar, low salt)

4 tbs sesame oil

1 thumb-sized piece ginger, grated

2 tbs honey or rice bran syrup

3 tbs soy sauce

pinch of chilli flakes

Simple steps:

Season the pork steaks well by rubbing with salt and pepper. Heat a non-stick pan over a medium heat and drizzle a little olive oil into the pan. Fry the steaks for 6 minutes on one side then turn once. Fry for a further 2 minutes on the other side then squeeze the juice of half a lime over the top of the steaks, remove from the pan and leave to rest for 2–3 minutes.

While the pork is cooking on side one, add the peanut butter, sesame oil, ginger, soy sauce, honey, chilli flakes, lime zest and remaining juice, along with four tablespoons of water, to a pan and heat gently, stirring every 30 seconds or so.

Steam the broccolini for 2–3 minutes then drain and season with a little salt and pepper and a drizzle of olive oil and transfer to a serving dish. Pan fry the garlic and carrots in a separate pan for 2–3 minutes. Add the noodles along with the peanut sauce and toss well. Slice the pork into strips and add to the noodles along with any juice from the pork. Serve with spring onions and crushed peanuts.

TOP TIP:

Double up on the ginger and peanut sauce and make a large batch. Store in a jar, then allow to cool and store in the fridge, ready for when you want to make this again.

GOOD TO KNOW:

Take my advice and use chopsticks to help slow you down while eating this. It's dangerously tasty and it's the only thing that worked for me ...

* Need this recipe a little lighter?
Simply reduce the olive oil 1 tbs (20ml) olive oil = 165 calories

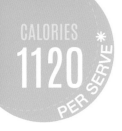

Dirty Crumbed Mexican Burger with Charred Corn

(SERVES 2)

Say hello to greatness people! You'll want to savor every bite of this loaded chicken burger. It's huge in the flavor department and wickedly simple.

You will need:

- 2 chicken breasts, butterflied
- ½ cup white flour
- 3 eggs, whisked
- 1 cup panko breadcrumbs
- 4 tsp Mexican spice mix
- 2 corn cobs
- 1 lime, zested and juiced
- 2 tbs yoghurt
- 1 tbs sriracha sauce
- 2 white burger buns
- 2 handfuls spinach
- 1 large tomato, sliced
- 2 slices cheddar cheese
- 3 tbs extra virgin olive oil

Simple steps:

Preheat the oven to 200°C (390°F) and place two large pieces of greaseproof paper on a chopping board. Place each chicken breast onto the paper and on its side and carefully slice along the breast with a sharp knife creating a large pocket. Continue slicing into the chicken until you are able to open it up but without slicing all the way through.

Lay the chicken breast out flat then place another piece of greaseproof paper on top of each breast. Using a rolling pin start rolling the chicken breast forwards and backwards, increasing the size of the chicken. Continue until the chicken breast is roughly 1-cm thick (0.4 in) across. Repeat steps with the other piece.

Place the flour in a bowl, the eggs in another bowl and the breadcrumbs in a third bowl. Add 2 teaspoons of Mexican spice to the flour and 1 teaspoon to the breadcrumbs and mix well while still keeping them separate.

Dip the chicken into the flour then into the egg wash, coating it well, then finally into the breadcrumbs. Then go back through the egg wash and finally through the breadcrumbs.

Drizzle a good amount of olive oil into a frying pan and fry the chicken over a medium heat for 2 minutes then turn over for another 2 minutes. Place the crumbed chicken onto an oven tray and roast for 10–12 minutes, ensuring the chicken is white all the way through before removing.

While the chicken is cooking place the corn in a pan of boiling water and cook for 3 minutes. Drain and dry the corn then fry in a pan with a little olive oil. Once the corn starts to char add the rest of the Mexican spice and coat the corn. Add half the lime juice then remove from the pan, taking care not to burn the spices.

Mix the yoghurt with the rest of the lime juice along with a good squeeze of sriracha sauce and spread onto the base of the burger bun. Add spinach leaves, tomato then the crumbed chicken. Add a slice of cheese and some more sriracha yoghurt.

TOP TIP:

For an easy life you can prepare the chicken in advance, right up to coating it in breadcrumbs, then wrap it in cling film and store it in the fridge for 2–3 days.

*Need this recipe a little lighter?
Simply reduce the olive oil 1 tbs (20ml) olive oil = 165 calories

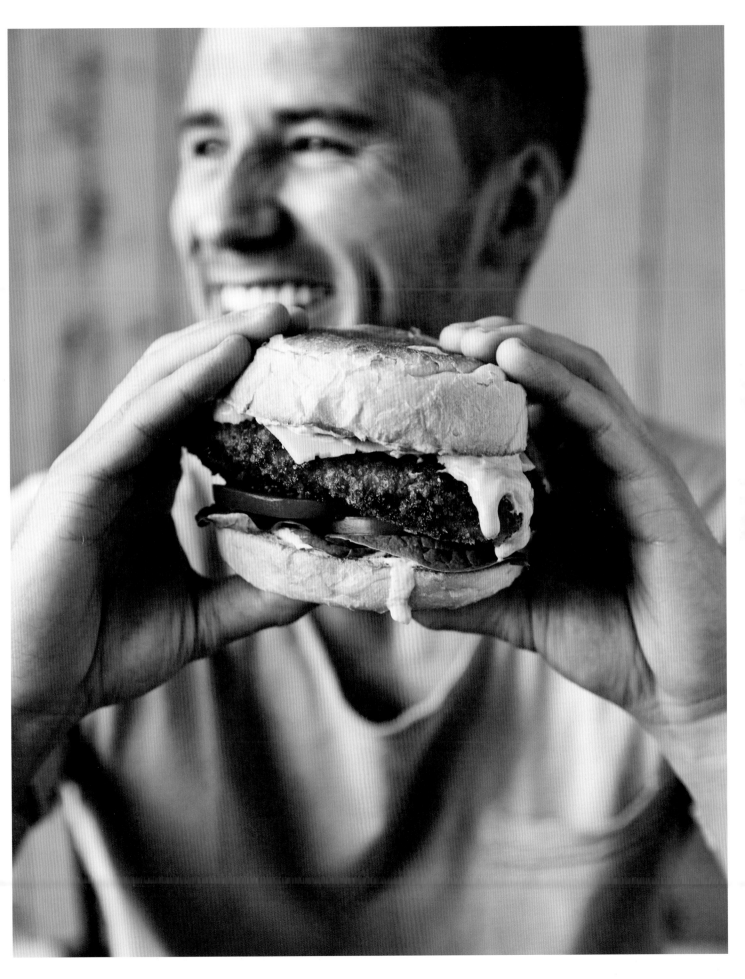

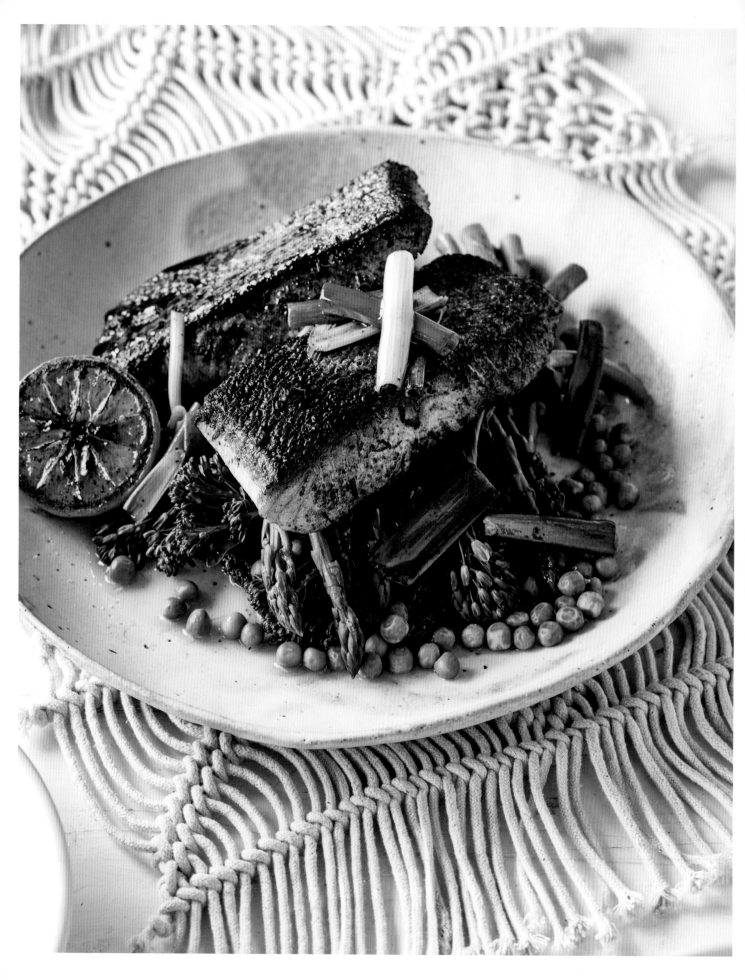

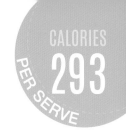

Crispy Cajun Salmon and Super Greens

(SERVES 2)

If you've never tried Cajun spice with salmon, you are in for a real treat. Cajun spice adds an exciting blend of zesty, spicy and savory flavor to take this salmon to a different level.

You will need:

- 2–3 tsp Cajun spice
- 2 salmon fillets (skin left on)
- 1 lime, zested
- 1 bunch broccolini
- 2 cups frozen peas
- 1 bunch asparagus
- ½ bunch spring onions (scallions), finely sliced
- extra virgin olive oil
- salt and pepper

Simple steps:

Heat a non-stick pan over a medium heat and drizzle a little olive oil into the pan. Rub the Cajun spice mix into the salmon along with a good pinch of salt. Pan fry skin side down for around 3–4 minutes. You are aiming to cook the fish around 60% through on the skin side before turning it over. Turn onto the flesh side and cook for another 2 minutes then turn onto the sides and cook for another minute each side. Once cooked squeeze half a lime over the top and remove from the pan to rest.

While the salmon is frying on the skin side, bring a pan of salted water to the boil and cook the broccolini, peas and asparagus for 2–3 minutes then drain and drizzle with a little olive oil.

Squeeze lime juice into a large serving dish and a good drizzle of olive oil, salt and pepper. Add the greens so the dish and toss through. Serve the salmon fillets on top and garnish with spring onions.

GOOD TO KNOW:

This dish is the perfect balance of high protein, omega 3s and fibrous super greens which provide a good dose of antioxidants, vitamins and minerals.

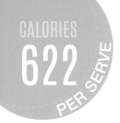

Mustard Rubbed Flank Steak with Creamed Leeks

(SERVES 2)

Super lean, full of flavor, and most importantly cheap, the flank is a great cut of beef for feeding a large family. Once tenderized you'll think it's a high-end cut and when paired with creamed leeks and spinach it'll blow your socks off.

You will need:

- 2 large flank steaks
- 1 tsp hot mustard
- 1 large leek, finely sliced
- 2 garlic cloves, finely diced
- ½ bunch fresh thyme, leaves picked
- 4 tbs crème fraîche
- 3 tsp wholegrain mustard
- 4 large handfuls spinach
- 10–12 button mushrooms
- 3 tbs extra virgin olive oil

Simple steps:

Preheat the oven to 200°C (390°F). Tear off a sheet of baking paper and place it on a chopping board. If you have a tenderizing mallet use this but if not, a rolling pin will do just fine. Lay the steak on the baking paper and hit it all over for about a minute or so. This will soften the fibers, making it juicer when you're eating it, and it will also flatten the steak to speed up the cooking time.

Heat a non-stick pan over a medium heat and add a good drizzle of olive oil. Season the steak well by rubbing salt and pepper over both steaks. Pan fry the steaks, turning every minute for 4 minutes for a 1 cm (0.4 in) thick steak. Transfer to an oven tray and roast in the oven for 4–5 minutes, then once cooked spread some hot mustard over the top and leave to rest for at least 3–4 minutes but do not wash the pan.

Drizzle a little more olive oil in the steak pan and fry the leeks, garlic and thyme. Fry for 2–3 minutes and then add the crème fraîche and wholegrain mustard. Add the meat juices released from the steak to the leeks as this is valuable flavor. Add the spinach, then once softened adjust the seasoning and spoon into a serving dish. Slice the steak and arrange on top of the creamed leeks. If there are any extra steak juices spoon these back over the top of the steak.

TOP TIP:

Flank steak is also fantastic to cook on a BBQ – try marinating for a few hours in some chopped garlic, fresh thyme, lemon rind and olive oil.

GOOD TO KNOW:

Red meat is a great source of **iron, zinc and vitamin B12.**

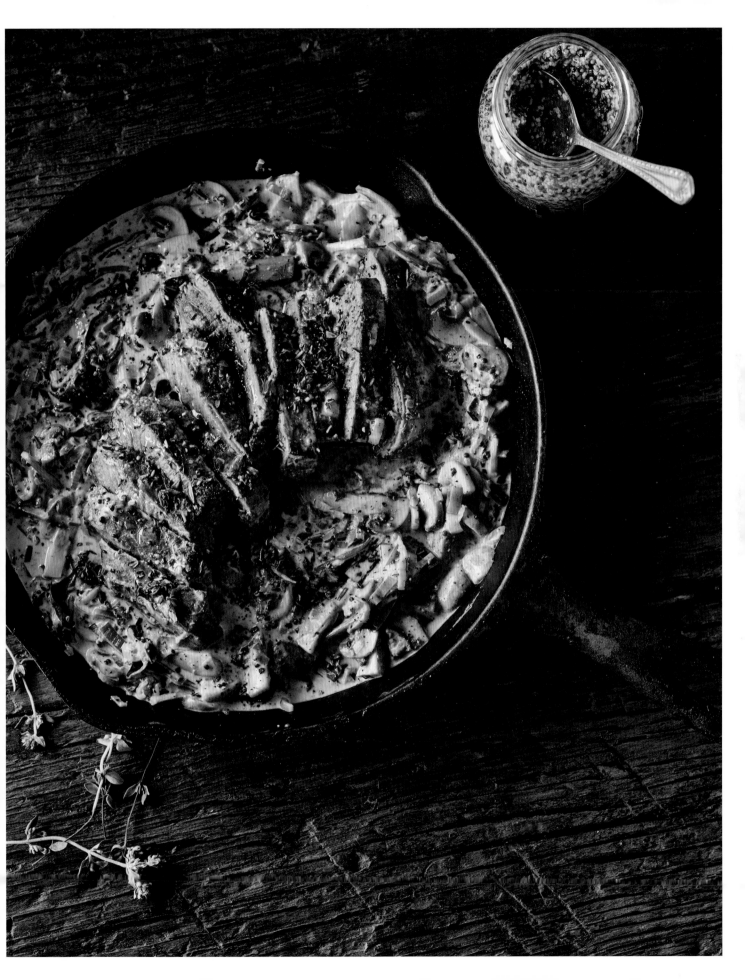

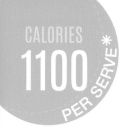

Maple and Soy Salmon Poke

(SERVES 2)

I almost turned into a poke bowl during my recent trip to Hawaii, it was all I ate.
All you need is the freshest fish, a bunch of crunchy vegetables
and a wicked dressing to make one of the healthiest bowls of food on the planet.

You will need:

250 g (8.8 oz) microwave brown rice

1 large carrot, grated

1 apple, finely sliced

1 cup cooked edamame beans

½ a cucumber diced

2 skinless salmon fillets, diced

2 large nori sheets

2 tbs sesame seeds

2 large spring onions (scallions), finely sliced

Maple and soy dressing:

3 tbs olive oil

2 tbs maple syrup

1 tbs soy sauce

2 tbs apple cider vinegar

1 garlic clove, finely diced

black pepper

Simple steps:

To build your poke bowl heat the rice in the microwave for the instructed time then spoon into a serving bowl. Add the sliced carrot, apple, edamame beans and cucumber around the side leaving a space in the middle.

In a clean jar combine the maple and soy dressing ingredients. Screw the lid on and give it a good old shake.

Add the diced salmon to a small bowl and pour over the dressing, mixing well. Arrange the salmon in the middle of the bowl and tip any excess dressing over the top of the salad.

Break up the nori sheets into small pieces and sprinkle over the top along with the sesame seeds and spring onions.

TOP TIP:

This poke bowl works brilliantly with raw tuna, or if you like your meat, add some sliced cooked chicken or beef as that works well too.

GOOD TO KNOW:

The omega-3 contained in salmon is essential for **good brain function.** Aim to eat fish two to three times a week, keeping an eye on the mercury content.

* Need this recipe a little lighter?
Simply reduce the olive oil 1 tbs (20ml) olive oil = 165 calories

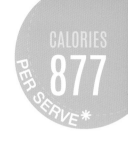
'Too Easy' Naked Burrito Bowl

(SERVES 2)

If you are anything like me, you love a Mexican burrito but hate that sluggish feeling afterwards. I've tied together everything you'd expect in a loaded burrito but tweaked it to leave you feeling guilt-free, but most definitely satisfied.

You will need:

2 chicken breasts, sliced into strips

3 tsp Mexican spice mix

1 lime, zested

1 large tomato, finely diced

½ a 400 g /113 g (14 oz) tin black beans

½ a red onion, finely diced

1 tsp smoked paprika

½ avocado

1 baby gem lettuce, sliced

½ bag shredded coleslaw mix (red cabbage, white cabbage, carrots)

100 g (3.5 oz) plain tortilla chips

chilli sauce (sriracha is my favorite)

3 tbs extra virgin olive oil

salt and pepper

Simple steps:

Throw the chicken into a bowl, add the Mexican spice mix and massage the spice into the chicken with your fingers.

Heat a pan on the stove over a medium heat and add a drizzle of olive oil. Fry the chicken for 3–4 minutes each side, turning regularly. Once cooked squeeze half the lime juice over the top and remove the pan from the heat but leave the chicken in the pan.

Mix the chopped tomatoes, black beans, red onion and smoked paprika in a small bowl and add a good pinch of salt and pepper and squeeze in the rest of the lime juice. Mash the avocado together in another small bowl and add a drizzle of olive oil, and a pinch of salt and pepper.

You can arrange your burrito bowl however you like, but I like to add the lettuce and the shredded cabbage to the bottom of the bowl, then add the sliced chicken along with the juice from the pan. Then arrange the Mexican beans and the avocado around the side along with a few, OK more than a few, tortilla chips. I also like to hit it with some spicy chilli sauce, but if it's not for you then ignore this step.

TOP TIP:

The thinner you slice the chicken the quicker it will cook, which leaves you more time to eat some extra tortillas! Just joking, but not really …

* Need this recipe a little lighter?
Simply reduce the olive oil 1 tbs (30ml) olive oil = 165 calories

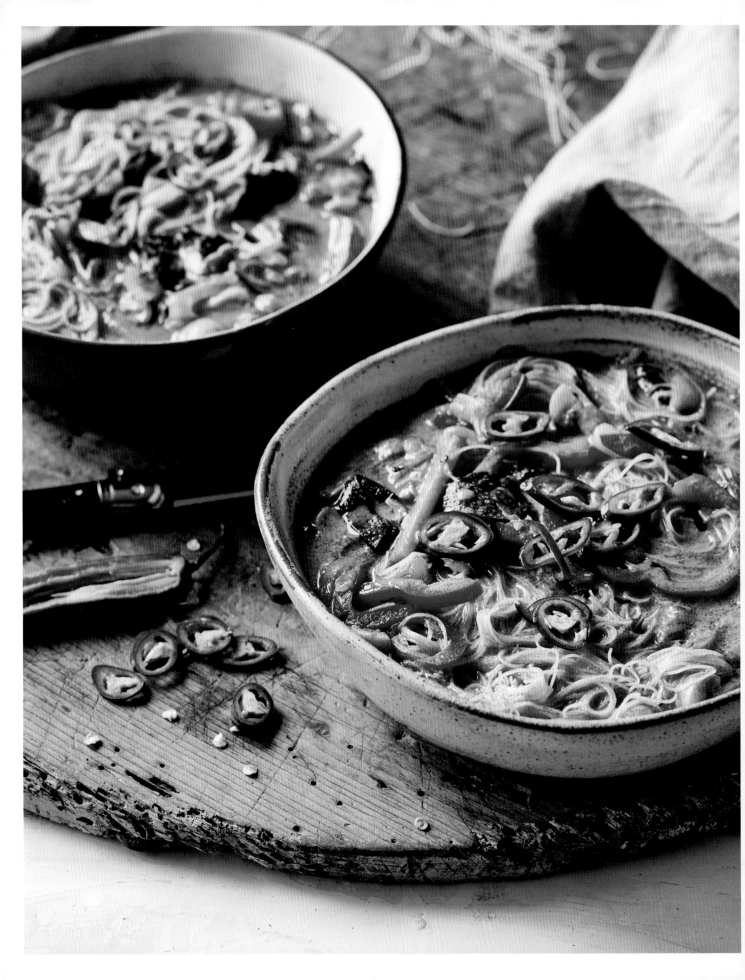

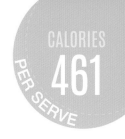

Spicy Thai Noodle Soup

(SERVES 4)

Ahh the humble noodle soup; guaranteed to put a smile on your face as soon as you have your first slurp. Infused with Thai aromatics and with the added bonus of throwing everything into one pot, it's made my list of must-cook soups!

You will need:

1 red onion, finely diced

2 garlic cloves, finely diced

1 large carrot, finely sliced

8 button mushrooms, quartered

1 bunch fresh basil, stalks finely chopped

3 tbs Thai red curry paste (as spicy as you like)

1 tbs fish sauce

1 lime, zested and juiced

1 red capsicum (bell pepper), finely sliced

400 ml (13.5 fl oz) tin coconut milk

500 ml (17 fl oz) chicken stock (reduced salt)

250 g (8.8 oz) packet vermicelli rice noodles

sesame oil to drizzle

pinch of chilli flakes

3 tbs extra virgin olive oil

Simple steps:

Heat a large non-stick pan over a medium heat with a good drizzle of olive oil. Fry the onion, garlic, carrots, mushrooms and basil stalks (finely chopped) until soft, saving the leaves for later. Add the Thai curry paste to the pan and stir on the heat for a minute or two. Add the fish sauce, lime zest, capsicum and coconut milk then reduce the heat.

In a separate pan, bring the chicken stock to the boil then add to the vegetables. Bring the soup back to the boil then turn the heat down to a simmer.

Put the noodles in a large bowl or dish and cover with lukewarm water for 3–4 minutes to soften, then drain.

Right before removing the pan from the heat, add the noodles and basil leaves and mix well. Serve each portion with a drizzle of sesame oil and a pinch of chilli flakes

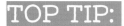 TOP TIP:

Be prepared for the flavor to intensify overnight, so make a large batch and get stuck in

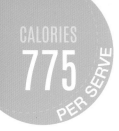

Firey Spaghettini Arrabbiata with Roasted Garlic

(SERVES 2)

Perfect pasta every time with authentic Italian flavors, that's made up almost entirely from your cupboard staples? Now you are talking my language! The chilli provides a welcoming smack in the chops, so for those spice lovers out there this dish is for you.

You will need:

150 g (5 oz) cherry tomatoes

3 whole garlic cloves, still in their skin

2–3 red chillies, finely sliced

1 bunch fresh basil, stalks finely chopped

1 ½ tbs white wine vinegar

400 g (14.5 oz) tin chopped tomatoes

200 g (7 oz) spaghettini

50 g (1.7 oz) parmesan cheese

½ lemon

3 tbs extra virgin olive oil

salt and pepper

Simple steps

Preheat the oven to 200°C (390°F), place the cherry tomatoes and garlic cloves (still in their skins) onto a small tray, drizzle with a little olive oil and roast for 15 minutes.

Heat a large non-stick pan over a medium heat and drizzle a little olive oil into the pan. Once hot fry the chillies, removing the seeds if they are very hot, but I like to take the risk. Add the finely chopped basil stalks, season with salt and pepper and fry for a few minutes until soft. Add a splash of vinegar to help balance the flavor then after about 30 seconds add the tinned tomatoes and bring to the boil then reduce the heat to a simmer.

While the sauce is simmering, cook the pasta in a large pan of salted boiling water. The spaghettini will only take 9–10 minutes. Make sure you cook it 'al dente' (with a little bite still left in the pasta), remembering it will continue to cook once you take it off the heat. Add a few spoons of pasta water to the arrabbiata sauce. The starch in the water helps loosen the sauce a little, plus you'll feel like a real Italian doing it.

Remove the tomatoes and garlic from the oven. Carefully squeeze the garlic out of the skins (the flesh will be really hot) then roughly chop, add to the sauce and stir.

Drain the pasta once it's cooked and add to the sauce. Give it a good toss in the pan then grate parmesan over the top. Add some torn basil leaves and serve. Top with roasted cherry tomatoes, extra parmesan, a good squeeze of fresh lemon juice along with a drizzle of good quality olive oil and black pepper.

TOP TIP:

Like every pasta dish this is super yummy eaten cold, making it a great dish to take to work as a leftover lunch. Feel free to add some cooked chicken if you're looking for a little extra protein.

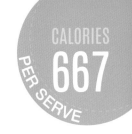

Bagged Barramundi with Curried Cauliflower Puree

(SERVES 2)

Creamy, comforting cauliflower puree that's been hit with some punchy spice,
is just the pairing to a meaty fish like barramundi.

You will need:

- 2 barramundi fillets
- 1 thumb-sized piece of ginger, finely sliced
- 1 lemon, half juiced and half sliced
- 1 large spring onion (scallion), roughly chopped
- 1 cauliflower head, cut into small florets
- 1 tbs butter
- ½ cup milk or coconut milk
- ½ onion, finely chopped
- 2 cloves garlic, finely chopped
- 3 tsp curry powder
- 4 large handfuls spinach
- 3 tbs extra virgin olive oil
- salt and pepper

TOP TIP:

To get ahead, simply get to the stage of wrapping the fish in the bag then store in the fridge. Pull it out of the fridge 5 minutes before you plan on cooking to allow it to come to room temperature then bake. I'll sometimes prep it to this stage before work in the morning.

GOOD TO KNOW:

Barramundi is a great source of **protein** and cooking it this way keeps it super soft, moist and full of flavor.

Simple steps:

Preheat the oven to 190°C (375°F). Place two large sheets of baking paper on your kitchen bench. Place the fish in the middle of each piece of paper. Season well with salt and pepper, then arrange the ginger on top of the fish along with a few slices of lemon. Sprinkle over the spring onions and give each piece of fish a good drizzle of olive oil.

Fold the edges of the paper up to the middle and wrap tightly, sealing in the fish and creating a tight bag. It doesn't have to look pretty but you'll get the best results with no holes in the bag so the fish can steam properly. Place the bags onto an oven tray then into the oven for 12–15 minutes depending on the thickness of your fillets. Remember that once you remove the fish from the oven it will continue to cook.

While the fish is cooking, steam the cauliflower florets in a steamer basket or colander with a lid over a pan of boiling water. Steam for 5–6 minutes or until soft. Gently heat the butter and milk in a small pan.

Pan fry the onions, garlic and curry powder in a little olive oil, seasoning with a good pinch of salt and pepper. Add the steamed cauliflower and toss. Carefully spoon the curried cauliflower into a blender along with the hot milk and butter and blend. Adjust the seasoning.

Place the spinach in the same colander you used for the cauliflower and steam for 60 seconds, then drizzle with a little olive oil and top with cracked black pepper and fresh lemon juice.

Serve the baked barramundi on top of the spinach with a generous serving of curried cauliflower puree.

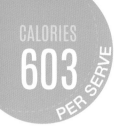

'Old School' Beef Rotolo with Burst Tomatoes

(SERVES 2)

I first tried beef rotolo when I traveled to Italy and was instantly obsessed: the creamy garlic, herb and sun-dried tomato ricotta stuffed inside the tender beef steak was so tasty. And the best news is you can get really creative with your fillings and choice of meat, or even vegetables.

You will need:

1 punnet cherry tomatoes

1 medium red onion, quartered

2–3 tbs balsamic vinegar

2 garlic cloves, grated

6–8 sun-dried tomatoes finely sliced

4 tbs ricotta cheese

2 beef topside fillets or flank, fillets bashed out

2 handfuls spinach

cooking twine or string

3 tbs extra virgin olive oil

salt and pepper

Simple steps:

Preheat the oven to 180°C (350°F). Put the cherry tomatoes, onion, salt and pepper, balsamic vinegar and a good drizzle of olive oil in a small oven dish and mix well with your hands. Place in the oven on the bottom shelf and roast for 12–15 minutes.

Mix the garlic, sun-dried tomatoes, a little olive oil, a pinch of salt and pepper and the ricotta cheese together in a bowl. Lay the steaks onto a sheet of baking paper then spread the ricotta generously over each piece. Place the spinach leaves neatly on top and roll the steak from one end. Tie the ends fairly tightly with two pieces of string to ensure the filling doesn't fall out when you cook them. You can tie another piece around the middle if you like.

Fry the beef rotolos in a non-stick pan with a little olive oil for 2–3 minutes, turning every so often, then place into an oven tray and roast for 8–10 minutes.

Serve a beef rotolo on a bed of the burst tomatoes.

TOP TIP:

This is another dish to prepare in advance and leave in the fridge. Remember to take it out five minutes before you plan on cooking, then pan fry and oven roast. Delicious!

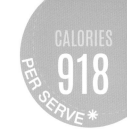
'Tasty As' Chicken Burger with Tarragon Crème Fraîche

(SERVES 2)

Come on! I mean if this isn't making your mouth water then I don't know what will. Stacked up high with layers of sweet beetroot, a chargrilled chicken patty, melted cheese and tarragon-hit crème fraîche it's a combo worth shouting about.

You will need

- 300 g (10 oz) chicken mince
- 1 red onion, half finely diced half finely sliced
- 1 garlic clove, grated
- 1 tsp dried oregano
- 1 bunch fresh tarragon, roughly chopped
- 2 tbs crème fraîche
- 2 soft burger buns (wholemeal optional)
- 1 baby gem lettuce, leaves picked
- 2 cooked beetroot, sliced
- 4 slices strong cheddar cheese
- 3 tbs extra virgin olive oil
- salt and pepper

Simple steps:

Place the mince, diced onion, garlic, oregano, half the tarragon and a good pinch of salt and pepper in into a large mixing bowl. Using your hands, get in there and give it a good mix up. Mold into large patties by starting with a ball of mince then pushing and shaping the mince using your palms to create two patties. Ensure they are both roughly the same size and thickness, about 2–3 cm (0.75 in) is good.

Heat a griddle pan over a high heat and drizzle a little olive oil into the pan. Fry the burgers for about 3–4 minutes each side then finish for a final minute on each side to get some real color going. If you don't have a griddle pan use a normal pan, or a BBQ will work even better for that flame-grilled taste. Once cooked all the way through remove the burgers from the pan and allow to rest for 2 minutes.

While the burgers are cooking mix the rest of the tarragon with the crème fraîche and season with a little salt and pepper. Place the buns under the grill and color slightly, then start to build your burger. Place a little crème fraîche on the bottom of the bun then add the lettuce, a slice of beetroot, burger, cheese and sliced onions. Top with another few slices of beetroot and some extra lettuce. Spread a generous spoon of crème fraîche onto the lid of the bun and place on top of the burger.

TOP TIP:

This isn't a first-date advised meal for those looking to play it cool. The sauce will go everywhere, but that's OK because what it lacks in being easy to eat it makes up for in deliciousness.

GOOD TO KNOW:

Make a load of patties in advance; they're great served with a salad or rolled into meatballs and served in a rich tomato sauce.

* Need this recipe a little lighter?
Simply reduce the olive oil 1 tbs (20ml) olive oil = 165 calories

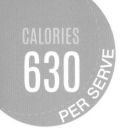

San Choy Bau

(SERVES 2)

Oh my goodness, I swear san choy bau should translate to 'little boats of heaven'. With crunchy lettuce cups filled with spicy mince it's seriously addictive. Say goodbye to Chinese food being a one-off because you'll want to eat this dish again and again.

You will need:

- 2 garlic cloves, grated
- 1 thumb sized piece of ginger, grated
- 1 red chilli finely sliced
- 300 g (10 oz) extra lean pork mince
- 1 tsp oyster sauce
- 3 tbs soy sauce
- 3 tsp sesame oil
- 2 large spring onions (scallions), chopped
- 1 bunch coriander (cilantro)
- 8–10 lettuce cups
- 1 handful peanuts, roughly chopped
- 2 tbs extra virgin olive oil

Simple steps:

Heat a large non-stick pan over a high heat, drizzle a little olive oil into the pan then fry the garlic, ginger, chilli and pork mince for a few minutes. Add the oyster sauce, soy sauce and sesame oil then turn down the heat until the pork mince is cooked.

Add the spring onions and coriander to the pork mince and stir. Spoon the mince into the lettuce cups and top with peanuts. Get ready to get messy!

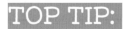

TOP TIP:

Great for an entree or side dish at a party or a bit of a lighter bite at dinner.

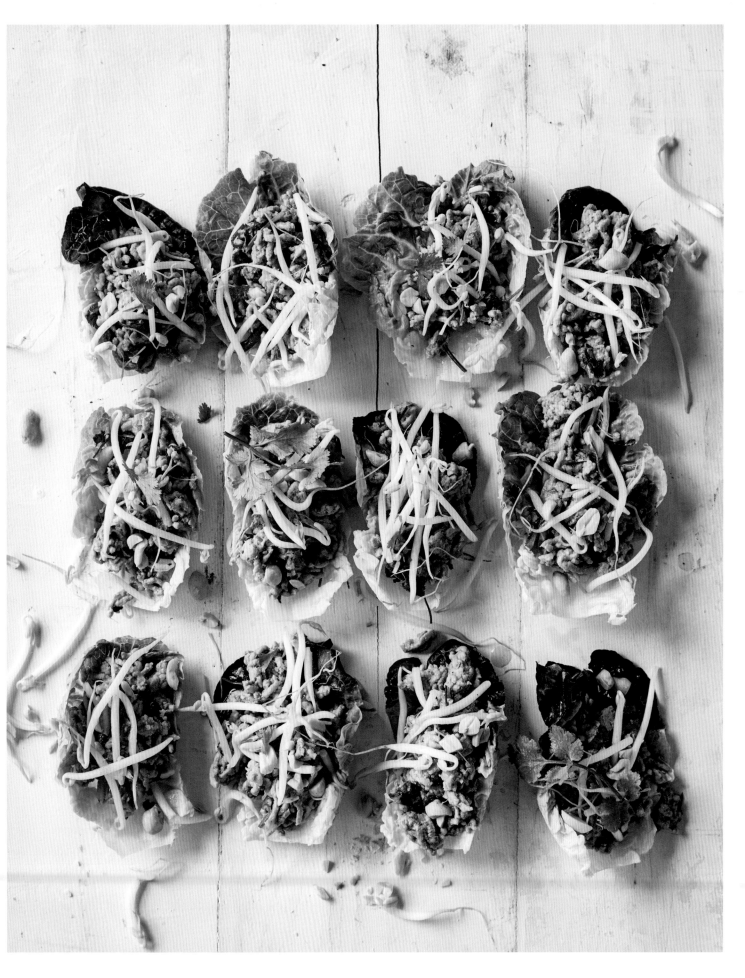

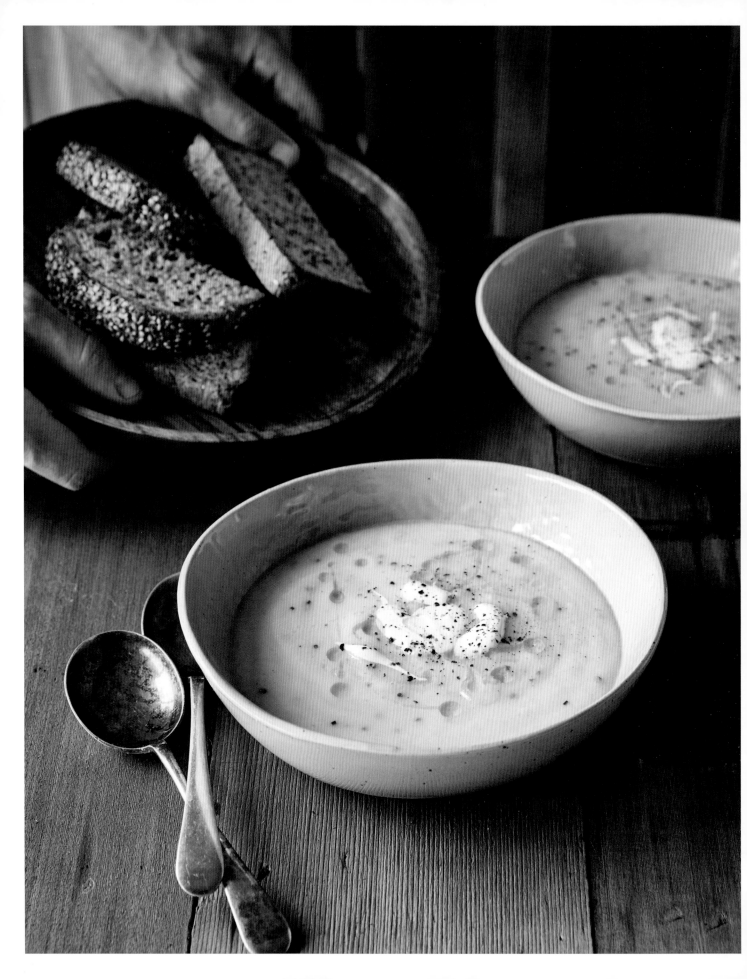

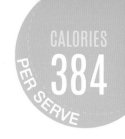
Cauliflower and Chive Soup with a Crusty Slice

(SERVES 4)

Soup in 20 minutes? Absolutely! Soups are super-quick to make, locking in the valuable vitamins and nutrients, and cauliflower and chive makes for such a great pairing.

You will need:

1 white onion, finely diced

2 garlic cloves, crushed

2 celery stalks, finely diced

2 medium-sized potatoes, finely diced

1 litre (33 fl oz) vegetable or chicken stock

1 large head of cauliflower, cut into florets

1 bunch chives, finely chopped

2 tbs crème fraîche

4 slices wholemeal bread

3 tbs extra virgin olive oil

salt and pepper

Simple steps:

Heat a large pan over medium heat and drizzle in some olive oil. Fry the onion, garlic and celery until golden brown then add the potato. Season well with salt and pepper.

Boil the stock in a separate pan and add to the vegetables. Bring to the boil then turn down to a simmer. After simmering for 3–4 minutes add the cauliflower florets and cook for 4–5 minutes or until the cauliflower is soft.

Remove from the heat once all the vegetables are cooked then blend straight away with either a stick blender or a stand blender. Be very careful when using a stand blender not to fill the jug too full. I like to place a tea towel over the top of the lid to prevent any hot liquid from spilling out.

Return the soup to the saucepan, add the chopped chives and give it one final stir then serve with a spoon of crème fraîche, a drizzle of olive oil, some cracked black pepper and a side of bread.

TOP TIP:

Dicing up your veg into small pieces means it'll take less time to cook and retain more flavor and valuable nutrition. Soup freezes really well so get ahead and store in 1–2 serve containers ready for when you're in need of a quick lunch or dinner.

GOOD TO KNOW:

Cauliflower is low in calories so it's a great choice if you are looking for something light but full of goodness. It's also an excellent source of vitamin C when eaten raw in salads.

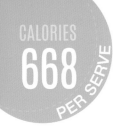
Cumin Rubbed Pork, Griddled Baby Gem and Pomegranate

(SERVES 2)

If you haven't tried charred lettuce before you are in a for a real treat; it's honestly a thing of beauty and when loaded with succulent spiced pork and sweet pomegranate seeds, oh my goodness, the taste is magic.

You will need:

- 2 pork steaks
- 2 tsp ground cumin
- 1 pomegranate
- 4 baby gem lettuce, quartered
- 2 tbs honey
- 1 tbs apple cider vinegar
- 50 g (1.7 oz) feta cheese, crumbled
- 2 tbs extra virgin olive oil
- salt and pepper

Simple steps:

Season the pork steaks well with salt, pepper and cumin spice, rubbing it all over and pressing it well into the meat. Leave to one side, bringing them up to room temperature.

Place the pomegranate on its side and slice in half. Holding it seed side down over a bowl, whack the skin with a metal spoon and the seeds should fall into the bowl. Remove any pith that ends up in the bowl. Drain off the juice and leave to one side as you will need this later.

Heat a griddle pan over a medium heat, although if you don't have one a regular non-stick pan will be fine. Drizzle a little olive oil into the pan and fry the pork steaks for 6 minutes on one side then turn over and fry for another 2 minutes, then remove from the pan and leave to rest for a final 2 minutes.

Tip out the oil from the pan and give it a little wipe then add a little fresh olive oil. Char the baby gem lettuce quarters in the pan and season. Once they start to get a little color drizzle a tablespoon of honey over the top then remove from the heat.

Drizzle some olive oil into a large dish then add a couple of tablespoons of fresh pomegranate juice, the rest of the honey and the apple cider vinegar. Add the lettuce and toss through the dressing. Slice the pork steaks and lay on top of the lettuce then finish with pomegranate seeds and crumbled feta cheese.

GOOD TO KNOW:

Pomegranates are among the healthiest fruits on the planet, containing high amounts of **antioxidants.**

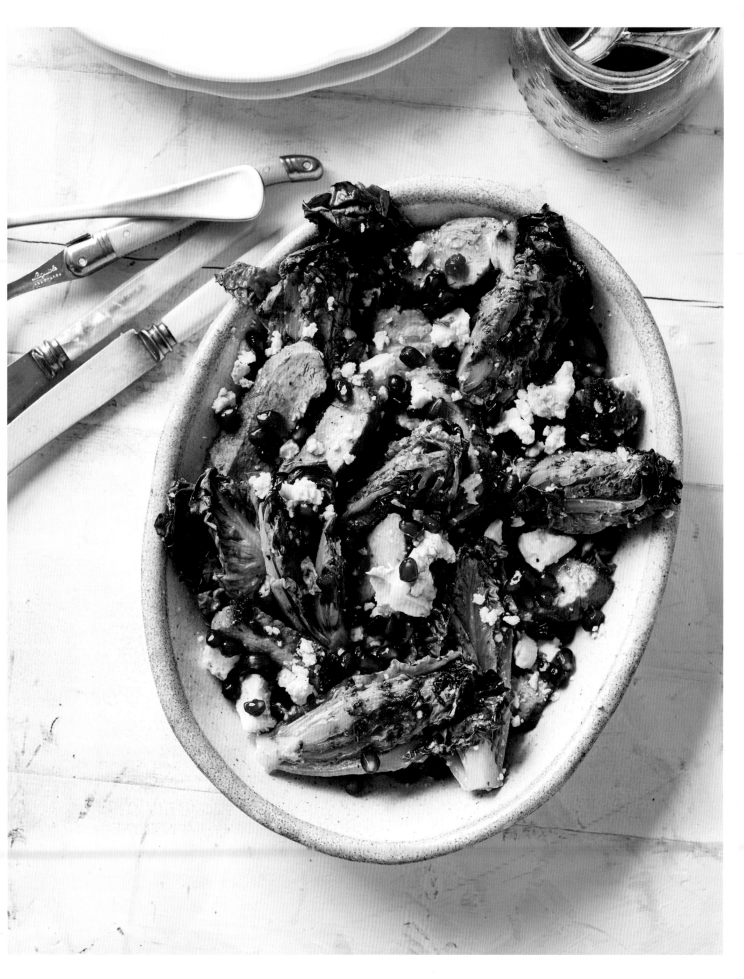

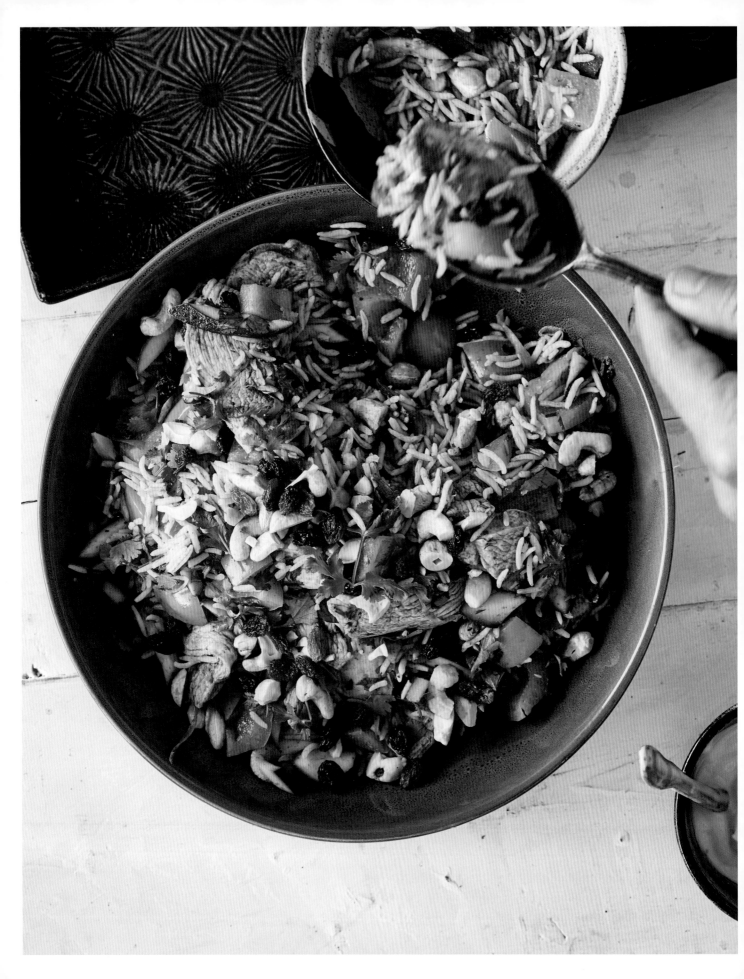

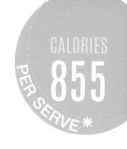

Harissa Chicken Stir Fry

(SERVES 2)

Skip the takeout, chicken stir fry has to be one of the simplest dinners to prepare. It's top of the list when I want something quick and easy.

You will need:

- 2 chicken breasts
- 2–3 tbs harissa paste
- 1 red onion, finely sliced
- 8–10 button mushrooms, sliced
- 1 garlic clove, finely sliced
- 1 zucchini, sliced
- 1 red capsicum (bell pepper), finely sliced
- ½ bunch coriander (cilantro), roughly chopped
- 1 handful sultanas
- 2 tbs sour cream
- 250 g (8.8 oz) microwave basmati rice
- 1 lime, zested and juiced
- 3 tbs extra virgin olive oil

Simple steps:

Slice the chicken breast into strips and place in a large mixing bowl. Add the harissa paste and rub into the chicken with your hands.

Heat a large non-stick pan over a high heat and drizzle in a little olive oil. Add the onion, mushrooms and garlic and fry for 2 minutes. Carefully add the chicken and fry for 5–6 minutes. Add the zucchini and capsicum then once the chicken is cooked all the way through add the coriander and sultanas then remove from the heat.

Throw the bag of rice into the microwave and cook in accordance with the instructions on the packet then once ready split between two serving dishes. To pimp up your rice add the lime zest and fresh lime juice along with a pinch of salt and give it a good stir. Serve the chicken stir fry on top of the rice and finish with the sour cream, extra coriander leaves and sultanas.

TOP TIP:

Ensure all of your vegetables are prepared before you start cooking. The key to a good stir fry is **speed** and having everything ready to just throw into a pan makes things much easier.

* Need this recipe a little lighter?
Simply reduce the olive oil 1 tbs (20ml) olive oil = 165 calories

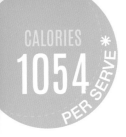

CALORIES
1054
PER SERVE *

Crumbed Barramundi with Orange and Watercress

(SERVES 2)

Crispy crumbed fish is a mid-week regular. Super light and much healthier than fried fish.

You will need:

- 1 cup panko breadcrumbs
- 1 lemon, zested then juiced
- 1 orange, zested then segmented
- 1 bunch parsley, half very finely chopped half roughly chopped
- 2 barramundi fillets
- 1 large bunch watercress
- ½ avocado, sliced
- 3 tbs extra virgin olive oil
- salt and pepper

Honey dressing:

- 1 lemon, juiced
- 1 tbs honey
- 4 tbs olive oil
- 2 tbs apple cider vinegar
- 1 garlic clove, finely grated or chopped

Simple steps:

Preheat the oven to 180°C (350°F). In a mixing bowl combine the breadcrumbs, the lemon and orange zest, finely chopped parsley and a good pinch of salt and pepper and mix well with your fingers.

Rub the barramundi fillets in olive oil then toss through the breadcrumbs, carefully packing the crumbs onto and around the fish. Don't worry if some of the herb crumb falls off the fish as you will add some more before you cook the fillets.

Line an oven tray with baking paper then place the fillets onto the tray. Add another drizzle of olive oil over the fillets then press the rest of the crumb onto the fish. Bake in the oven for 12–15 minutes depending on the size of the fillet.

While the fish is cooking put the honey-lemon dressing ingredients in a clean jar, screw the lid on and give it a good old shake.

Arrange the watercress on a large platter along with the rest of the parsley and scatter the orange segments and avocado slices over the top. Dress the leaves with the honey-lemon dressing and place the barramundi fillets on top. Sprinkle any crispy breadcrumbs that have fallen off while cooking over the salad for some extra crunch.

TOP TIP:

The barramundi fillets will continue to cook once you remove them from the oven, so I'd advise cooking them a little under and allowing the residual heat to cook them to perfection.

GOOD TO KNOW:

This is one super-healthy salad: the watercress is packed with nutrients particularly **vitamin K** while the avocado provides a good amount of healthy fats, which can help to lower cholesterol.

* Need this recipe a little lighter?
Simply reduce the olive oil 1 tbs (20ml) olive oil = 165 calories

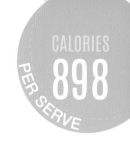
Garlic Chilli Prawn Linguine with Secret Butter

(SERVES 2)

Okay, so weeknights just got a little bit more interesting with this unbelievably moreish, linguine pasta. The secret butter adds a naughty little kick that you can add to pretty much anything.

You will need:

- 150 g (5 oz) unsalted butter at room temperature (don't worry, this makes several portions)
- 1 bunch parsley and stalks, finely chopped
- ½ tsp chili flakes
- 1 lime, zested and juiced
- 3 garlic cloves, grated
- 200 g (7 oz) dried linguini pasta
- 8–10 sun-dried tomatoes in oil, finely chopped
- 250 g (9 oz) cooked prawns
- 3 tbs extra virgin olive oil
- salt and pepper

Simple steps:

Add the softened butter to a mixing bowl along with half the chopped parsley, chilli flakes, salt and pepper, lime zest and grated garlic. Mix well with a spoon.

Spread a large sheet of greaseproof paper roughly 40 x 40 cm (15 x 15 in) on your kitchen top. Spoon the butter in the middle of the paper and shape into a rough sausage shape. Roll the paper over the top of the butter and fold it. Holding the ends tightly, roll the butter back and forth several times until you start to see a neat sausage shape forming. Fold in both ends and transfer to the freezer to set.

Cook the linguine in a pan of salted boiling water for 9–10 minutes depending on the thickness. Remember cooking it 'al dente' (firm to the bite) is the best way to enjoy pasta.

About halfway through cooking the pasta, heat a pan over medium heat, add a little of the sun-dried tomato oil along with the sun-dried tomatoes and finely chopped parsley stalks. After 2 minutes add the prawns and toss for 1 minute. Squeeze fresh lime juice over the prawns then quickly remove the pan from the heat.

Drain the pasta then add to the prawns and tomatoes with a touch of the pasta water to help loosen it up. Remove the butter from the freezer and slice into 3 x 1 cm (0.3 in) slices and add to the pasta. Give it a good toss and serve with a few extra slices of fresh lime.

TOP TIP:

The next time you want to use the butter, remove it from the freezer about 10 minutes beforehand to soften, otherwise you can soften it in the microwave but do this in stages so it doesn't completely melt.

GOOD TO KNOW:

The secret butter works amazingly well melted over steak, rubbed over sweetcorn or tossed through roasted vegetables.

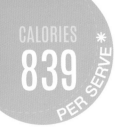

Roasted Roots and 'Beet It Up' Pesto

(SERVES 3)

I love this lazy recipe because all you have to do is simply throw all the veggies into one big tray and give them a damn good roasting – you don't even have to peel them! Plus, the natural sugars released when cooking the veg this way create little caramelized pieces of deliciousness.

You will need:

4 carrots, sliced

2 medium sweet potatoes, sliced

2 red onions, quartered

4 parsnips, sliced

8 garlic cloves, in their skin

6 tbs extra virgin olive oil

salt and pepper

'Beet it up' pesto:

2 handfuls pine nuts, toasted

3 cooked beetroot

50 g (1.7 oz) parmesan cheese

1 lemon, zested and juiced

Simple steps:

Preheat the oven to 200°C (390°F). Give the vegetables a good scrub to remove the dirt then top and tail all the vegetables and slice into even-sized pieces. Scatter on a large oven tray along with the garlic cloves, keeping them in the skins. Drizzle a generous amount of olive oil over the top of the veg along with a good pinch of salt and pepper and roast in the oven for 18–20 minutes.

While the vegetables are roasting, toast the pine nuts in a dry pan over medium heat until golden brown.

Halfway through roasting the vegetables remove four of the garlic cloves from the tray and squeeze out the flesh into a food processor. Add the beetroot, parmesan cheese, pine nuts (reserving some to use as a garnish), lemon zest, olive oil, and a twist of salt and pepper. Give it a good blend for about 15–20 seconds. I like to leave my pesto a little chunky as it adds some great texture to the vegetables.

Once the roasted vegetables are cooked, remove the rest of the garlic and squeeze out the flesh onto a chopping board. Roughly chop then carefully mix back through the vegetables. Spread the beetroot pesto over the bottom of a large serving dish and top with the roasted veg and extra pine nuts and some freshly squeezed lemon juice.

TOP TIP:

Double your 'beet it up' pesto portions and store a jar in the fridge for 2–3 days. Simply serve with vegetable sticks or crackers for a delicious snack.

GOOD TO KNOW:

Eating beetroot can help to keep the **liver** healthy and it's also a great source of vitamin C.

* Need this recipe a little lighter?
Simply reduce the olive oil 1 tbs (20ml) olive oil = 165 calories

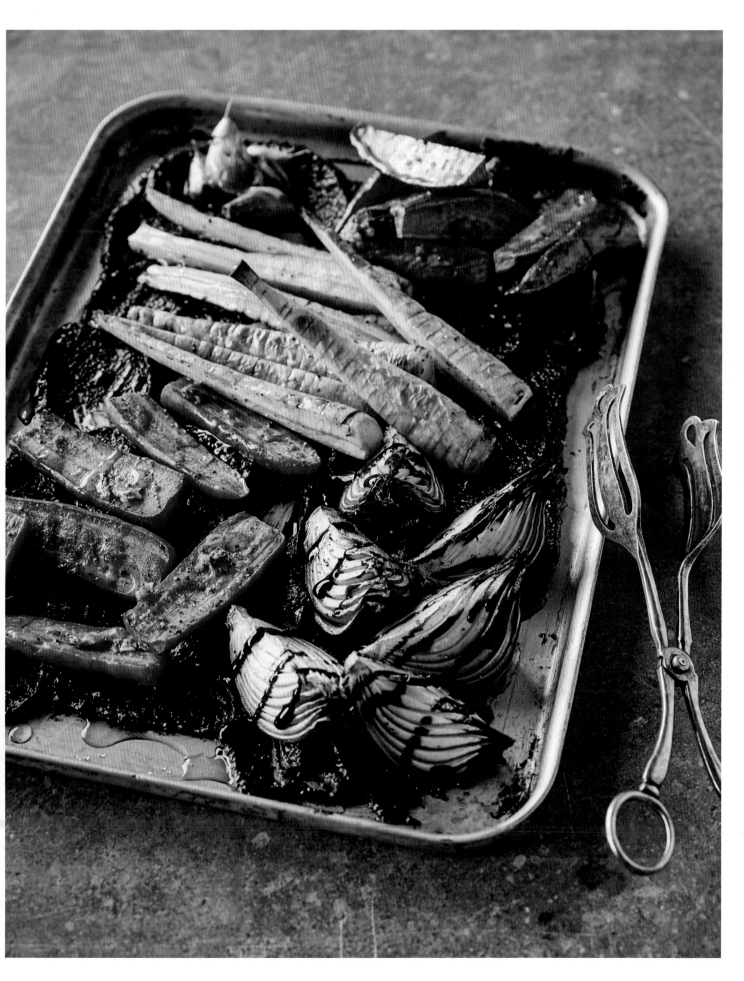

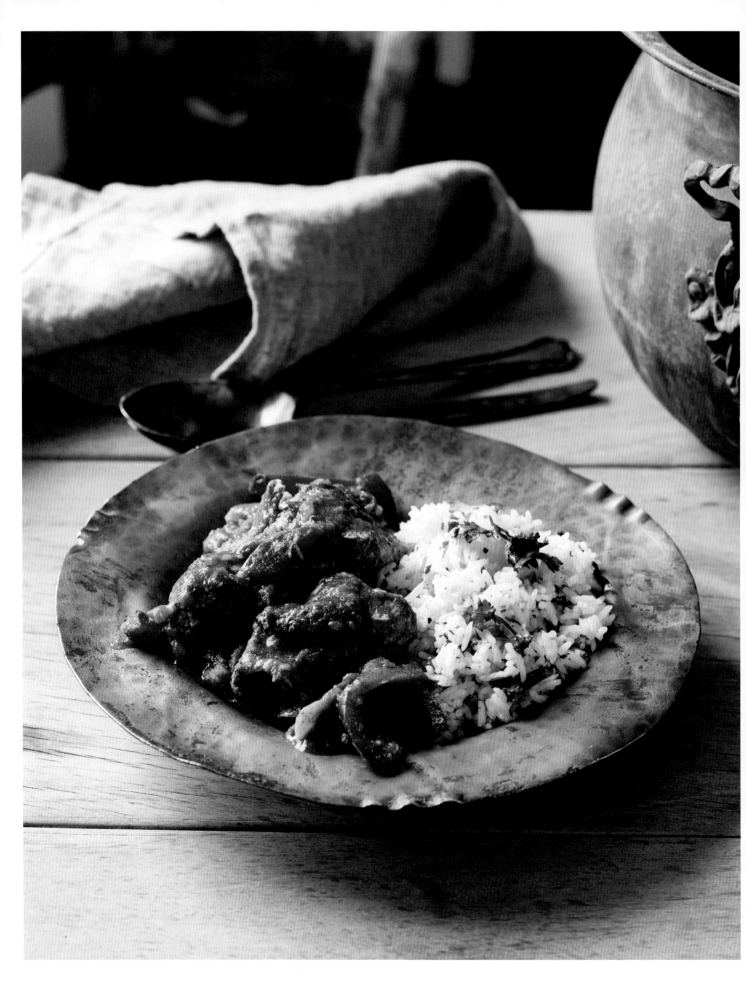

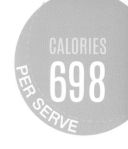

Indian Cheat's Chicken Tenders with Infused Rice

(SERVES 2)

These delicious strips of chicken can be knocked up quicker than you can order your takeaway, and I guarantee you won't be ordering anything else. Indian-inspired flavors without the hassle: you just can't beat these classic Indian spices!

You will need:

- 2 large skinless chicken breasts
- 1 red capsicum (bell pepper), finely chopped
- 2 medium tomatoes, finely diced
- 2 garlic cloves, finely crushed
- 2 tbs ground cumin
- 2 tbs curry powder
- 2 tsp paprika
- ½ tsp chilli flakes (optional)
- 250 g (8.8 oz) microwave basmati rice
- 1 bunch coriander (cilantro), roughly chopped
- 2 tbs extra virgin olive oil
- salt and pepper

Simple steps:

Preheat the oven to 220°C (430°F). Slice the chicken into thick strips and place in a bowl with the capsicum, tomato and garlic. Add the spices along with the chilli flakes if you like a little punch to your chicken. Drizzle olive oil over the top along with a good pinch of salt then massage together, ensuring every piece of chicken is well covered.

Spread the ingredients onto an oven tray and roast for 15–18 minutes. Ensure the chicken is white in the middle and cooked all the way through before removing. Once cooked remove the chicken and place on a plate and allow to rest for 2–3 minutes, leaving the vegetables on the tray.

Using a potato masher, mash the tomatoes, capsicum and garlic together. Once the veg starts to break down a little it's ready to spoon into a serving dish. Add the chicken to the dish, along with any resting juices and mix well.

Cook the rice in the microwave in accordance with the instructions on the packet then divide between two plates. Serve the chicken with a generous topping of tomato and capsicum sauce.

TOP TIP:

Leaving the chicken to marinate overnight will kick the intensity up another notch so if you are organized enough this is a great idea for a quick win.

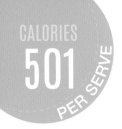

Crying Tiger and a Heap of Greens

(SERVES 2)

I first tasted this dish at a street market in Bangkok and, wow, it absolutely blew my mind. The heat hits you straight in the face and makes your eyes water as the name suggests, but it's strangely addictive If you like your spicy food, you'll love this.

You will need:

350–400 g (10.5–14 oz) eye fillet

1 tbsp soy sauce

1 tbsp fish sauce

2 bok choy, quartered

1 bunch broccolini

1 tbs sesame seeds

Crying tiger dipping sauce:

½ bunch coriander (cilantro), finely chopped (including stalks)

2 spring onions (scallions), finely sliced

1 birds-eye chilli, finely chopped

½ tsp chilli flakes

1 tbs oyster sauce

3 tbsp fish sauce

2 tsp honey

3 limes, juiced

2 tsp raw white rice (yes you read that right!)

extra virgin olive oil

TOP TIP:

If you buy a slightly larger fillet then stick to these cooking times: roast for 15 minutes per 500 g for medium rare and 20 minutes for medium, and remember to rest the meat for at least 5 minutes after removing it from the oven.

GOOD TO KNOW:

Beef is high in protein and a fantastic source of **zinc** and **iron** and vitamin **B12**, which helps maintain healthy cells in the body.

Simple steps:

Preheat the oven to 200°C (390°F). Put the meat in a dish and spoon over the soy sauce along with 1 tablespoon of fish sauce. Leave to marinate for a minute or two.

Meanwhile, finely chop the coriander stalks and add them to a small mixing bowl along with the spring onions, fresh chilli and flakes, oyster sauce, 3 tablespoons of fish sauce, honey and lime juice. Whisk everything together well.

Put the raw rice in a dry pan and toast over a medium heat for 2–3 minutes until it just starts to color. Tip into a mortar and pestle and give it a good bash. Add half to the crying tiger sauce and leave the rest to one side.

Drizzle a little olive oil in a pan and place over medium heat. Hold the fillet over the bowl for a few seconds to allow the sauce to drip off then very carefully place into the frying pan. The meat will spit a little at first so be careful! Fry for 1–2 minutes each side getting a really nice even sear. Wrap in tin foil and pour the juices over the top of the fillet then roast in the oven for about 10 minutes. Remove and leave to rest on a plate for 5 minutes.

Steam the bok choy and broccolini for 2–3 minutes. Slice the steak and spoon a little of the dipping sauce over the top then serve on the bed of greens and top with fresh coriander leaves, sesame seeds and the rest of the toasted rice.

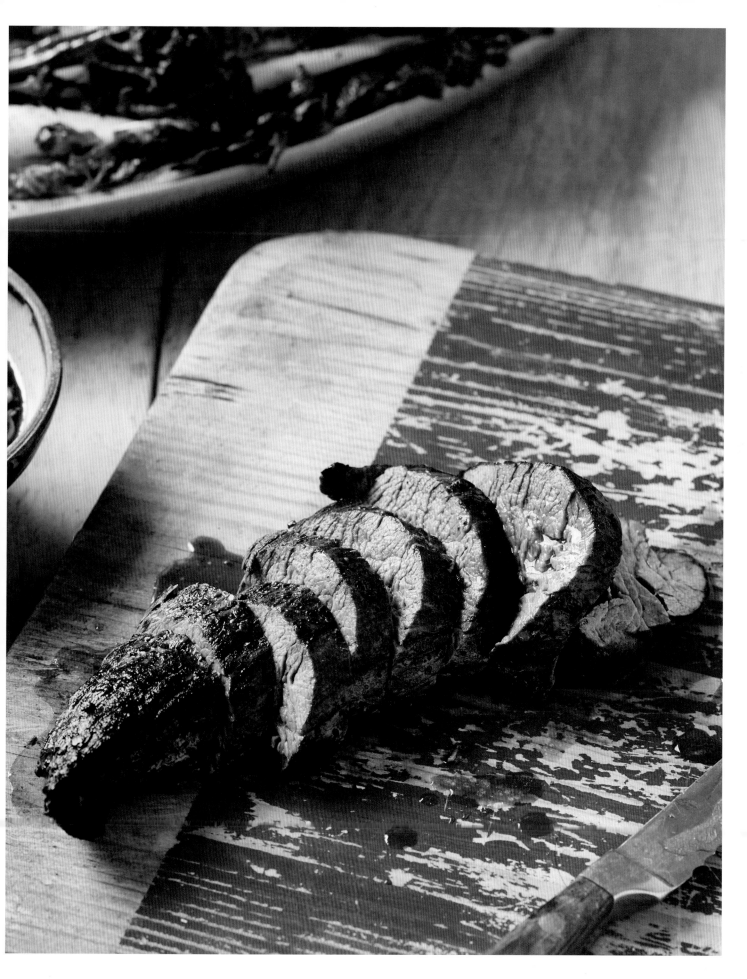

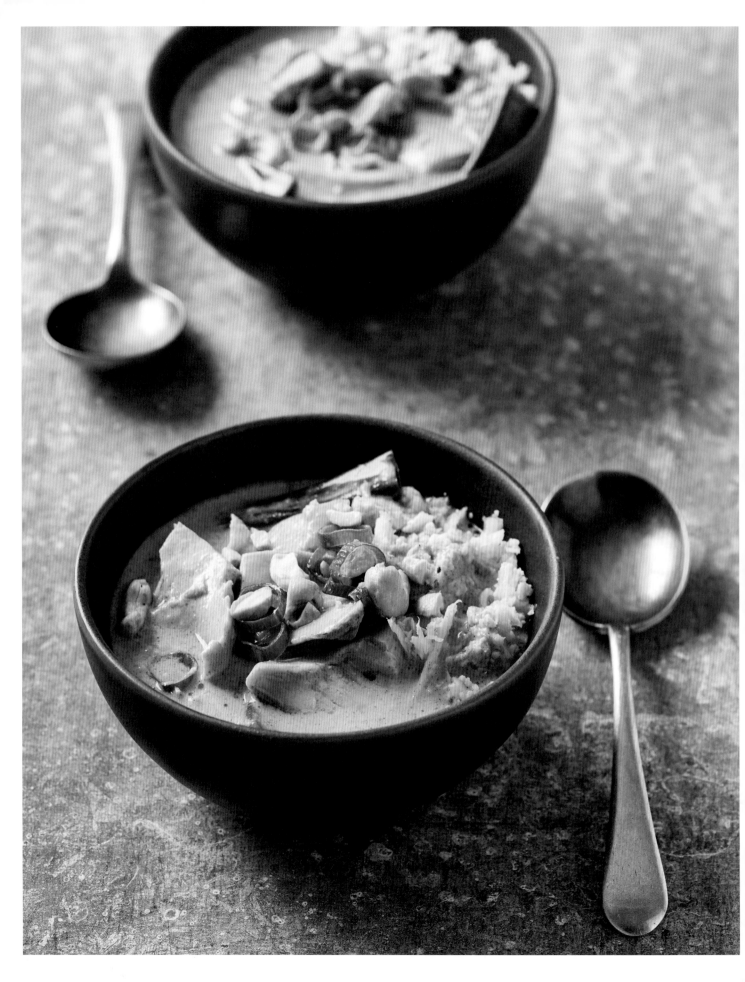

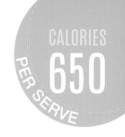

CALORIES
650
PER SERVE

Coconut Poached Salmon and Cauliflower Rice

(SERVES 2)

Gently poached in Thai aromatics, this rich coconut salmon broth is the ultimate feel-good food you'll want to make again and again. The broth is so tasty you'd be happy with a bowl just on its own.

You will need:

- 1 lemongrass stalk
- 1 tbs Thai red curry paste
- 1 lime, zested and juiced
- 2 spring onions (scallions), finely sliced
- 1 chilli, finely sliced
- 400 ml (13.5 fl oz) tin coconut milk
- 2 salmon fillets (skinless)
- 4 handfuls spinach
- 1 medium cauliflower, grated
- 1 small white onion, diced
- 2 garlic cloves
- 1 handful cashews, roughly chopped
- 3 tbs extra virgin olive oil

Simple steps:

Place the lemongrass onto a chopping board and bash with the back of a knife, splitting it a little to release the aromas. Transfer to a large pan along with the curry paste, lime zest, one spring onion, and the chilli. Pour in the coconut milk and mix everything together.

Gently bring the coconut milk to the boil then carefully add the salmon filets to the pan. Reduce the heat to a simmer for 4–5 minutes. Add the spinach, place a lid on the pan and remove from the heat leaving the salmon fillets in the hot coconut milk for another 4–5 minutes.

While the salmon is cooking, grate the cauliflower and leave to one side. Pan fry the onion and garlic in a little olive oil for 2 minutes then add the cauliflower and fry for another 2–3 minutes. Add a ladleful of the coconut milk the salmon has been infusing into the cauliflower then take the pan off the heat and squeeze in the juice of half a lime.

Toast the cashews in a dry pan over medium heat until golden. To serve, divide the cauliflower between the serving bowls or plates and flake the salmon over it. Ladle the coconut poaching milk over the top and finish with some toasted cashews and the rest of the spring onions.

TOP TIP:

Get ahead and grate the cauliflower in advance, ready to just throw into the pan.

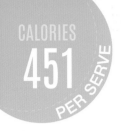

Lentil and Egg Dahl

(SERVES 4)

Lentils fill me with joy every time I eat them. It's great to have a break from meat knowing you're still getting a good portion of protein in. If you've never enjoyed lentils and eggs together then you are in for a real treat: they are a perfect meat-free option.

You will need:

1 cup dried red lentils

1 white onion, finely diced

2 garlic cloves, finely diced

2 celery stalks, finely diced

2 tsp curry powder

1 ½ tsp ground turmeric

500 ml (17 fl oz) vegetable stock

4 handfuls spinach

4 eggs

½ bunch fresh parsley, roughly chopped

2 wholemeal pitta breads

3 tbs extra virgin olive oil

salt and pepper

Simple steps:

Rinse the lentils under cold water and drain.

Heat a large non-stick pan over a medium heat and add a good drizzle of olive oil. Fry the onion, garlic and celery until soft. Add the curry powder and turmeric and fry for another minute. Add the lentils along with the vegetable stock and bring to the boil. Reduce to a simmer and cook for 15 minutes. Ensure the lentils are always covered with liquid while cooking so if they start to absorb too much of the stock just add a little water.

About 2 minutes before the lentils are cooked add the spinach. The lentils should be soft but still just holding their shape.

Boil a saucepan of water, then carefully add the eggs. I'd recommend doing this with a spoon and lowering them in one at a time so you don't crack the shell. Set a timer for 7 minutes for soft-boiled eggs and 9 minutes for hard-boiled eggs.

Fold some fresh parsley leaves into the lentils, taste and adjust the seasoning with salt and pepper. Once cooked peel the eggs and slice in half. Serve the lentils topped with soft-boiled eggs and a good drizzle of olive oil over the top, along with some toasted pitta breads on the side.

GOOD TO KNOW:

High in protein and **low in fat**, lentils are a rich source of **vitamin E**, which acts as an **antioxidant** in the body.

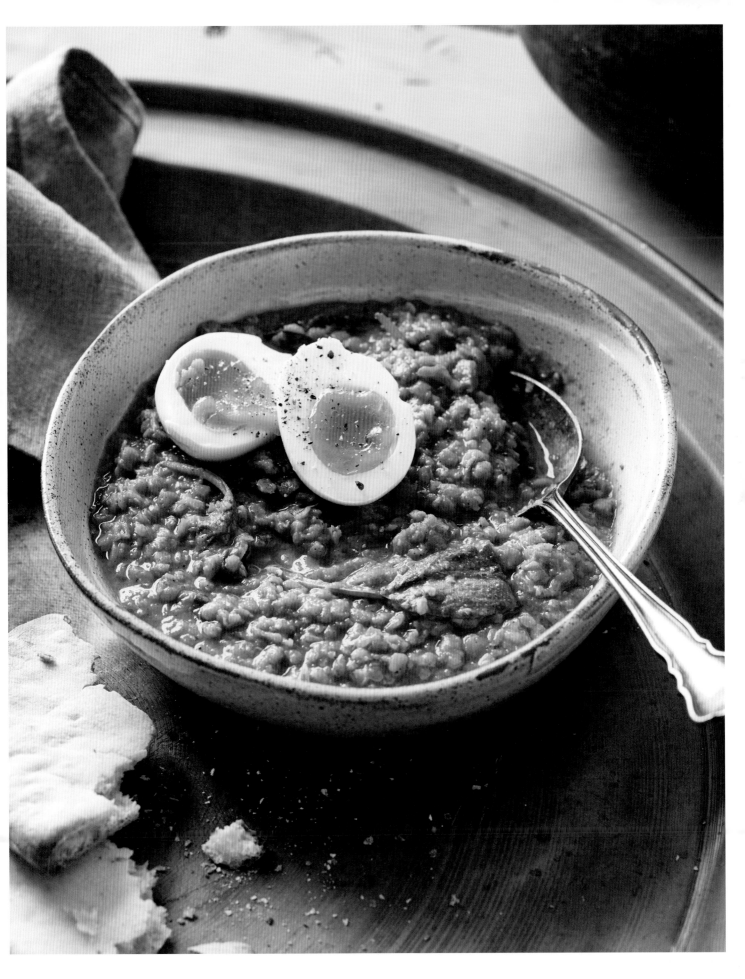

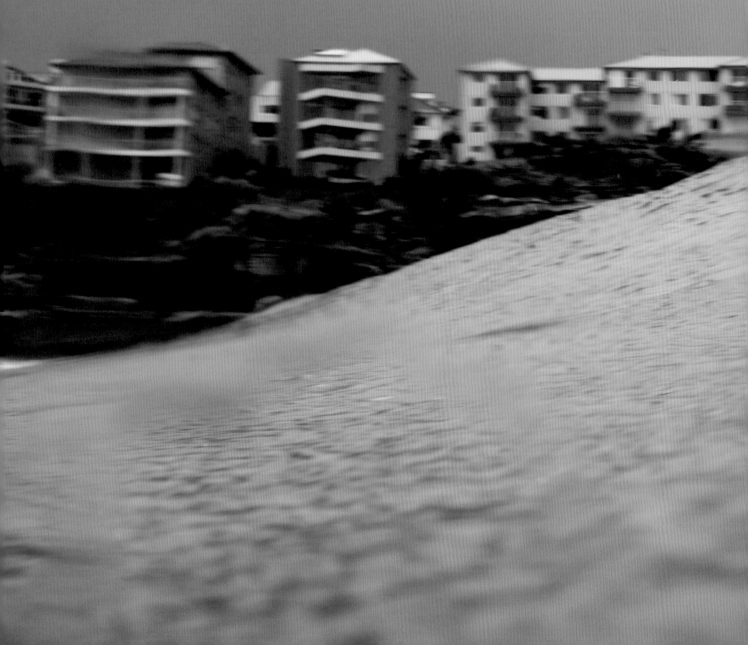

'Find something that motivates you,

because motivation
drives consistency
and consistency
is what get results'

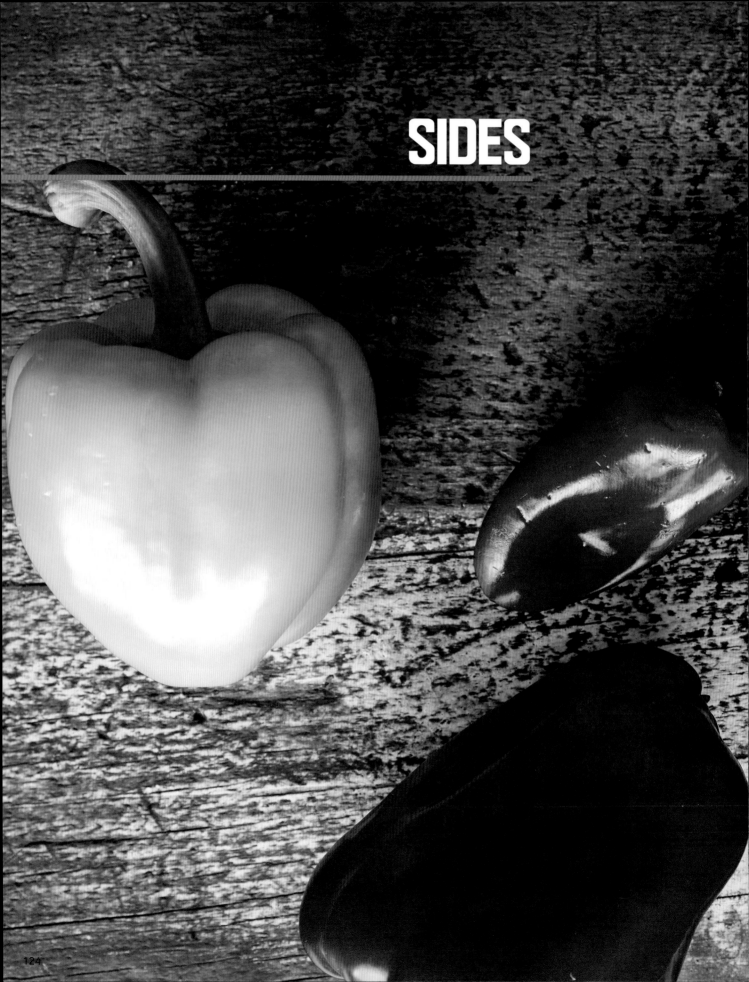

SIDES

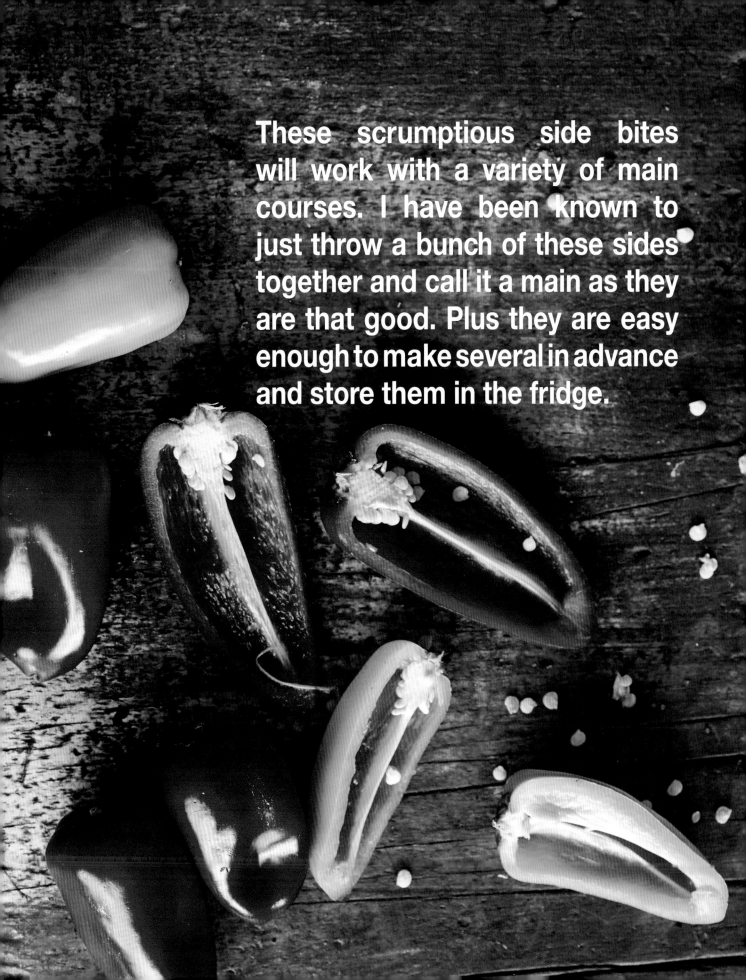

These scrumptious side bites will work with a variety of main courses. I have been known to just throw a bunch of these sides together and call it a main as they are that good. Plus they are easy enough to make several in advance and store them in the fridge.

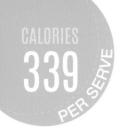

Garlic Broccolini With Roasted Almonds

(SERVES 2)

We all know broccoli is good for you, but it can get a little tough to eat. Broccolini on the other hand is a different story. Fresh, crunchy and with so many different dishes to add it to, this super green is a regular on my table.

You will need:

2 bunches broccolini

2 garlic cloves, very finely sliced

25 g (0.8 oz) parmesan cheese, grated

1 handful dry-roasted almonds, chopped

2 tbs extra virgin olive oil

salt and pepper

Simple steps:

Slice the ends off the broccolini. Boil quarter of a saucepan of water on the stove and place a steamer attachment or colander on top. Add the broccolini and place a lid on top. Steam for 2–3 minutes.

Meanwhile, heat a non-stick pan over a medium heat with a little olive oil. Add the garlic and fry until crispy – this won't take long so keep an eye on it. Once crispy tip the garlic onto some kitchen roll to remove some of the oil and leave to one side.

Drain the broccolini then add to the pan, season well with salt and pepper and give it a good toss. Grate parmesan cheese over the top and finish with almonds and crispy garlic.

GOOD TO KNOW:

Broccolini delivers a great dose of **vitamin C** and **vitamin K.** It also contains health-promoting plant compounds that have **anti-inflammatory** properties.

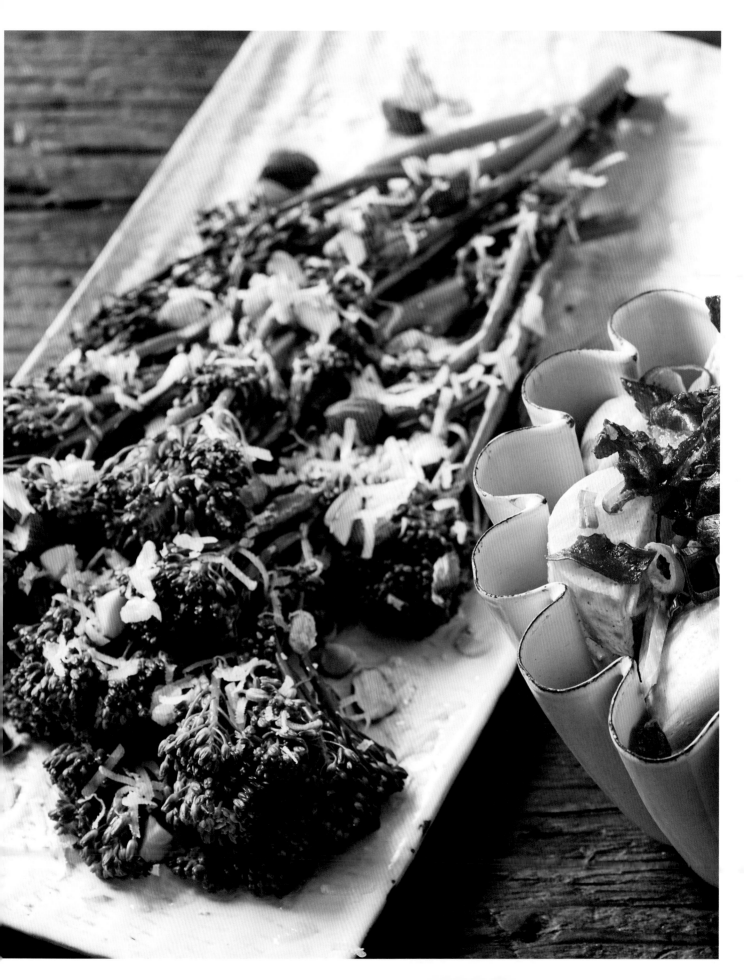

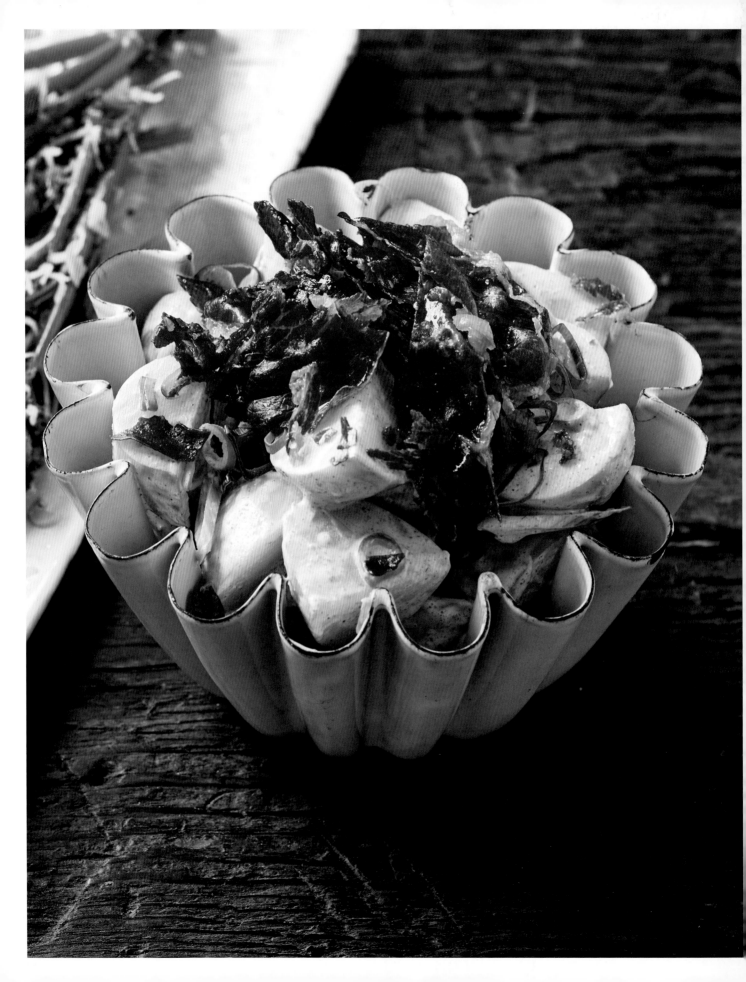

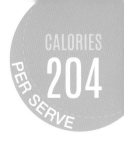

Bangin' Potato Salad

(SERVES 4)

Potato salad is an absolute game changer, and without a tub of mayonnaise in sight it's half the calories of the usually rich classic. Whether enjoyed at a BBQ or served alongside a beautiful piece of fish, potato salad will forever be on the menu.

You will need:

500g (17 oz) new or baby potatoes, halved

100 g (3.5 oz) Parma ham

4 tbs sour cream

1 lemon, zested

2 tsp ground cumin

2 large spring onions (scallions), finely diced

salt and pepper

Simple steps:

Preheat the oven to 200°C. Place the potatoes in a saucepan, cover with cold water and bring to the boil. Cook for 12–15 minutes until soft but still with a little bite to them. Rinse under cold water and then drain until bone dry.

Line a roasting tray with some greaseproof paper and lay the Parma ham on top. Roast in the oven for 10–12 minutes until crispy. Remove and transfer to a cooling rack to crisp up.

Meanwhile, put the sour cream in a bowl along with the lemon zest, cumin, spring onions and a good pinch of salt and pepper and mix well.

Tip the potatoes into a large serving dish and spoon over the sour cream then mix well. Break up the Parma ham with your fingers and scatter over the top.

GOOD TO KNOW:

Don't fear the yummy potato just because it's a carbohydrate, it's full of good stuff and surprisingly low in calories.

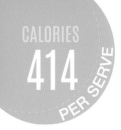
Mediterranean Tomato Salad with Balsamic Dressing

(SERVES 2)

I am so into this salad: it's quick, super fresh and guaranteed to brighten up any meal you serve it alongside. Don't be scared to mix up the tomatoes as they all provide different levels of sweetness and colors.

You will need:

½ punnet mixed cherry tomatoes sliced in half

1 small red onion, finely diced

2–3 large red and yellow tomatoes, sliced

110 g (3.8 oz) mozzarella

½ bunch basil

1 garlic clove, grated

2 tbs good quality balsamic vinegar

2 tbs extra virgin olive oil

1 tsp capers, chopped (optional but delicious)

salt and pepper

Simple steps:

Place the cherry tomatoes, onion and garlic in a serving dish. Season well with salt and pepper then mix together with your hands.

Arrange the sliced tomatoes around the cherry tomatoes, then tear the mozzarella cheese into small pieces, arrange over the top of the tomatoes and add the capers.

Put the balsamic vinegar and olive oil in a jar, screw the lid on tightly and give it a good shake. Spoon over the top of the tomatoes and finish with basil leaves.

GOOD TO KNOW:

Rich in nutrients such as **lycopene**, tomatoes have so many health benefits and could even help with our cardiovascular health. Happy days!

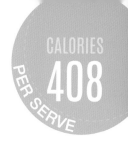

Hot Mexican Black Beans

(SERVES 2)

Load these guys into a soft taco, scatter over a salad or simply serve alongside a juicy steak.

You will need:

½ tin, 200 g (7 oz) black beans

½ tin, 200 g (7 oz) pinto beans

1 onion, diced

2 garlic cloves, grated

50 g (1.7 oz) feta cheese, crumbled

1 red birds-eye chilli, finely chopped

2 tsp smoked paprika

1 tbs tomato puree

1 lime, juiced

½ bunch coriander (cilantro), roughly chopped

2 tbs extra virgin olive oil

salt and pepper

Simple steps:

Rinse and drain the beans under cold running water. Heat a non-stick pan over a medium heat and drizzle in a little olive oil. Fry the onion, garlic and chilli for 2–3 minutes until soft. Add the smoked paprika and a good pinch of salt and pepper. Add the tomato puree along with 2–3 tablespoons of water then cook for 2 minutes. Add the beans and give the pan a good toss. After 2–3 minutes add the lime juice and the coriander then remove from the heat and crumble feta cheese over the top.

GOOD TO KNOW:

Black beans are a great source of nutritional fiber, protein and carbohydrates.

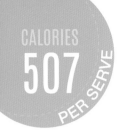

Super Cheesy
Broccoli and Potato Mash

(SERVES 2)

Mash potato wins the award for the ultimate comfort food in my opinion. Jazzed up with broccoli and loaded with cheddar cheese it's a bowl of deliciousness that pairs well with steak, chicken or even fish.

You will need:

100 g (3.5 oz) cheddar cheese, grated

200 g (7 oz) potatoes, chopped into small pieces (desiree, King Edward and sebago are ideal types for mashing)

1 head broccoli, cut into florets

25 g (0.8 oz) butter

1 tbs extra virgin olive oil

salt and pepper

Simple steps:

Put the potatoes in a saucepan with a good pinch of salt then cover with cold water. Place the pan on the stove and bring to the boil. Cook for 15–20 minutes depending on how small you have cut the potatoes.

Grate the cheese and leave it to one side (try not to eat all of this while you're cooking!). Bring a separate pan of water to the boil, then about 5 minutes before the potatoes are ready add the broccoli florets to the water and boil for 5 minutes.

Drain the broccoli and leave to one side. Also drain the potatoes well then place the lid back on the pan and give it a good shake, removing as much of the water as you can. The more water you remove the fluffier your mash will be.

Combine the potatoes and broccoli then using a potato masher give them a good mash. Add the butter and a good pinch of salt, pepper and a good drizzle of olive oil. Mash again until smooth. Finally fold in the cheddar cheese and serve immediately.

TOP TIP:

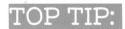

To reheat, simply place in a non-stick pan over a low-to-medium heat for 3–4 minutes stirring continuously.

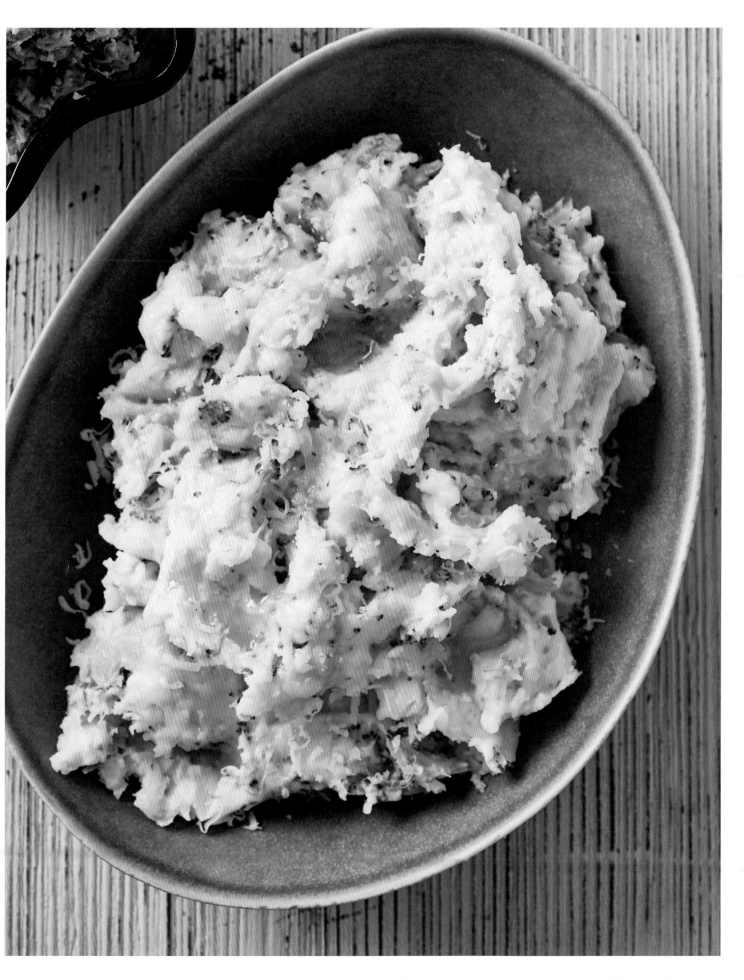

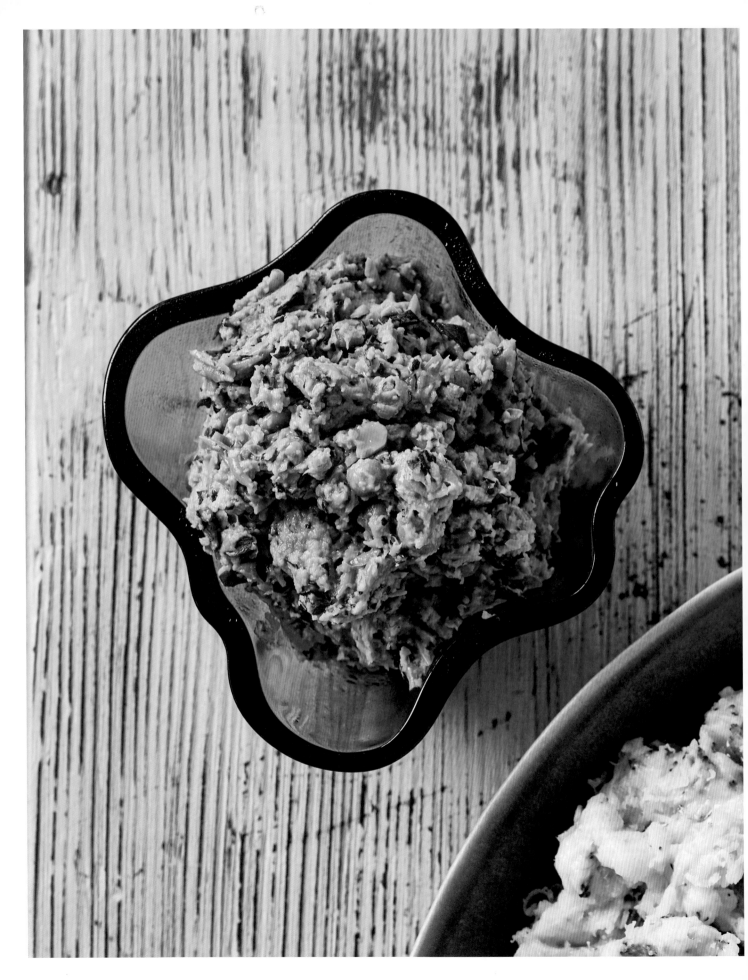

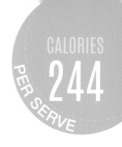

Smashed Minted Peas

(SERVES 2)

I used to hate mushy peas at school; overcooked and tasteless they were often pushed to the side of my plate. But I'm here to show you how to take the old school classic to a different level. Elevating them with mint and zingy lemon, these smashed peas are totally delicious and full of freshness.

You will need:

- 1 bowl frozen peas
- ½ bunch fresh mint, leaves picked
- 1 lemon
- 2 tbs extra virgin olive oil
- salt and pepper

Simple steps:

Steam or boil the peas for 3 minutes. Drain and transfer to either a metal mixing bowl or food processor. Add the mint leaves to the peas.

Pulse the peas using a stick blender or food processor for 20–30 seconds. Add a good squeeze of lemon juice along with a good drizzle of olive oil and a pinch of salt and pepper. Pulse for another 5 seconds then serve. I like to keep mine fairly chunky to add some texture.

GOOD TO KNOW:

Peas are rich in minerals such as **potassium, calcium** and **magnesium**.

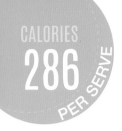

Cabbage Slaw with Balsamic Vinaigrette

(SERVES 4)

Light, colorful and super crunchy, cabbage slaw is the OG side that is welcome in my fridge anytime. I'll knock up a large bowl of this at the start of the week and enjoy it with some roast chicken breast or some baked fish. Yummo!

You will need:

½ red cabbage finely sliced

1 onion, finely sliced

1 pear, finely sliced

2 carrots, grated

1 apple, grated

Balsamic vinaigrette:

3 tbs balsamic vinegar

4 tbs extra virgin olive oil

1 tsp honey

2 tsp sesame seeds

pinch salt and pepper

Simple steps:

If you have a mandolin in the kitchen, you'll be able to slice the vegetables nice and fine, if not take your time by finely slicing the cabbage, onion and pear with a sharp knife.

Add the grated carrot and apple to a small bowl and mix together, then squeeze the juice from the carrot and apple into a bowl with your hands. Pour the juice into a glass and enjoy (it's delicious!).

Transfer the slaw mix to a large bowl.

To make the dressing, put the ingredients in a jar, screw the lid on tightly then give it a good old shake.

Spoon the vinaigrette over the top of the slaw just before you are about to serve.

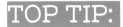
TOP TIP:

If you aren't planning on eating it straight away, leave it in the jar in a cool dry place.

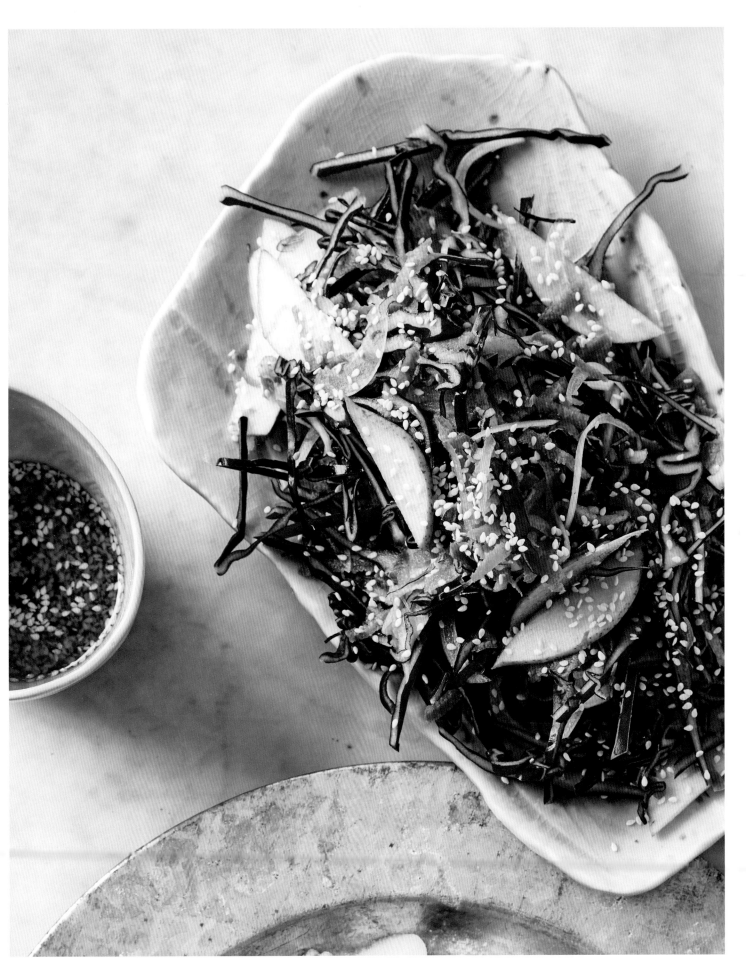

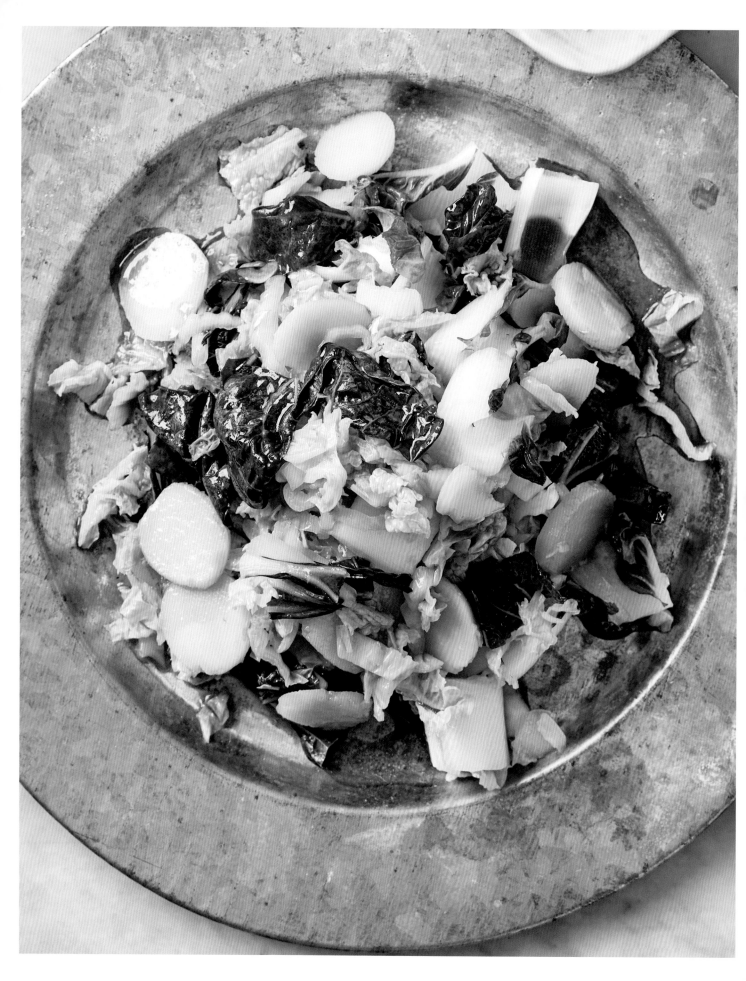

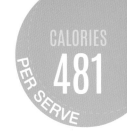
Asian Greens with Ginger, Honey and Soy

(SERVES 2)

Sometimes the best-tasting sides are the ones you have to fuss the least over.
Well it doesn't get much more fuss-free than shaking up some dressing and pouring
it over a big bowl of perfectly steamed healthy greens.

You will need:

2 tbs soy sauce

1 ½ tsp honey

2 tbs rice wine vinegar

4 tbs sesame oil

2 bok choy

½ a Chinese cabbage, finely sliced

1 garlic clove, finely sliced

½ a thumb-sized piece of ginger, finely sliced

225 g (8 oz) / 1 tin water chestnuts, sliced

1 tbs sesame seeds, toasted

Simple steps:

Add the soy, honey, rice wine vinegar and 2 tablespoons of sesame oil to a jar, then screw the lid on tightly and give it a good old shake.

Slice the bok choy in half lengthways, place in a steamer and steam for 1 minute. Add the Chinese cabbage and steam for another 2 minutes.

Pan fry the garlic and ginger in the rest of the sesame oil over a medium heat until lightly colored. Once cooked toss the Asian greens through the pan along with the water chestnuts, adding a good pinch of salt and pepper. Serve in a large dish and dress with the honey and soy dressing. Toast the sesame seeds in a pan with no oil for 2 minutes until golden and sprinkle over the top to finish.

TOP TIP:

To create your own steamer simply fill a deep saucepan one third full of water and place a large colander on top. Place the veg into the colander then place a lid on top.

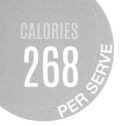

Mind-Blowing Chunky Guac

(SERVES 4)

Who doesn't love a good guac! Well I'm confident in saying this will be the best you've ever had. Creamy, show-stopping guac in less than 10 minutes that's perfect every time! You're welcome!

You will need:

- 2 ripe avocados
- 1 red onion, very finely chopped
- 2 medium tomatoes, finely chopped
- 2 garlic cloves, very finely grated
- 1 tsp chilli flakes
- 1 lime, zested and juiced
- 1 bunch coriander (cilantro), roughly chopped
- 2 tbs extra virgin olive oil
- salt and pepper

Simple steps:

Slice the avocados in half and remove the stones. Using a knife, carefully score into the flesh lengthways and then across. Grab a spoon and scoop out the flesh into a large mixing bowl. Using a potato masher mash the avocado until it starts to form a guacamole consistency. I like to keep mine lightly chunky and with a bit of texture. Add the red onion, tomatoes, garlic, chilli flakes, lemon zest and juice, a good pinch of salt and pepper and mix well. Top with some extra chilli flakes and a drizzle of olive oil.

TOP TIP:

Be generous with the salt and pepper seasoning. Avocado needs a little helping hand to bring out that delicious flavor. To prevent your guac from going brown drizzle a little olive oil over the top then tear off some cling film and spread it over the guac so it's in contact then refrigerate.

GOOD TO KNOW:

Full of **cholesterol-lowering healthy fats**, avocados are 'top of the tree' when looking to improve your health and are a great snack option any time of the day and night.

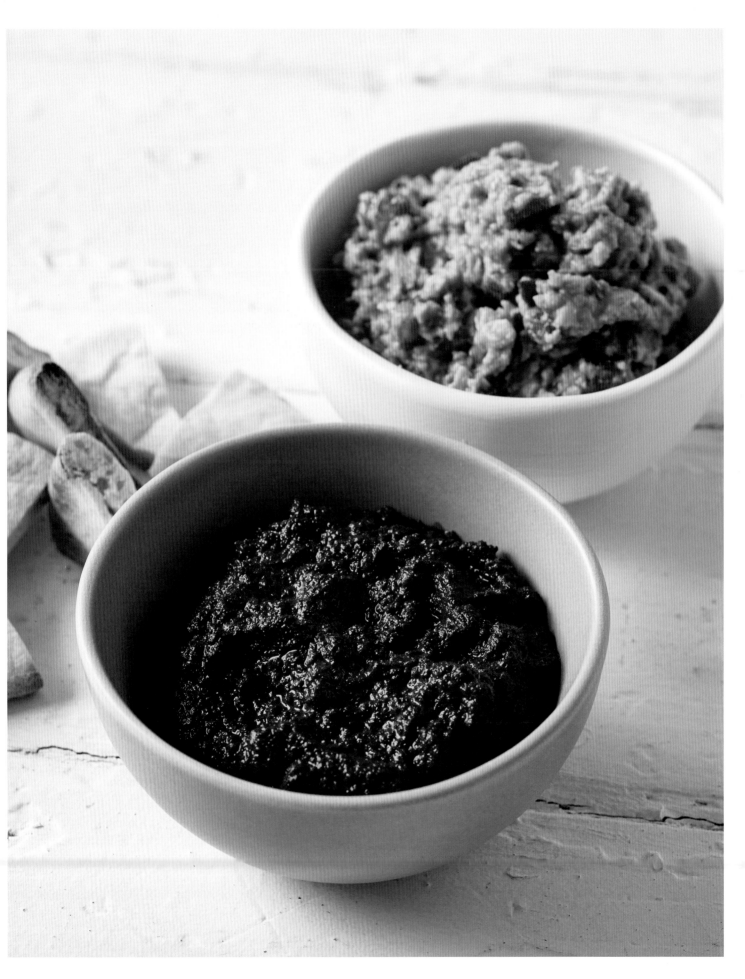

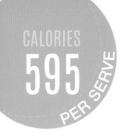

Zingy Beetroot and Cumin Dip

(SERVES 2)

I'll happily smother this onto some crusty bread with a side of wilted spinach and a squeeze of fresh lemon for a filling and nutritious lunch.

You will need:

4 cooked beetroot

2 garlic cloves, crushed

1 tsp ground cumin

6 tbs extra virgin olive oil

½ lemon, juiced

3 tbs natural yoghurt

salt and pepper

Simple steps:

Add the beetroot to a food processor along with the garlic, cumin, olive oil and lemon juice and pulse until smooth. Tip into a bowl, fold in the yoghurt and add a good pinch of salt and pepper.

TOP TIP:

Spread over toast and finish with some crumbled feta and dukkah spice and you've got yourself one tasty snack!

GOOD TO KNOW:

With links to potentially reducing blood pressure beetroot is the real deal. It's also packed with **fiber** so great for **gut health**.

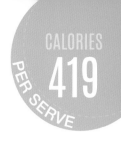

Creamy Sun-Dried Tomato Hummus

(SERVES 4)

Trust me when I tell you you'll never be buying
shop-bought hummus again, it's that good!

You will need:

1+½ tins chick peas / 600 g (21 oz)
   (garbanzo beans)

10–12 sun-dried tomatoes

2 garlic cloves finely chopped

1 tbs tahini, optional but delicious

½ bunch parsley chopped

1 tsp paprika

1 lemon

6 tbs extra virgin olive oil

salt and pepper

Simple steps:

Rinse and drain the chickpeas and place in a food processor along with the rest of the ingredients and blend until well combined. I like to leave a few chunky bits in my hummus for texture. Adjust the seasoning then scoop into a serving bowl.

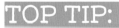

TOP TIP:

Cover with cling film and store in the fridge for 3–4 days. Serve with vegetable sticks or add to the top of a wicked salad for a high-protein hit!

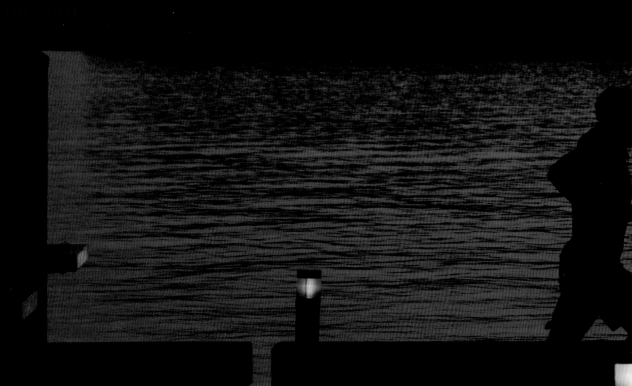

'Pick a form of exercise that suits you,

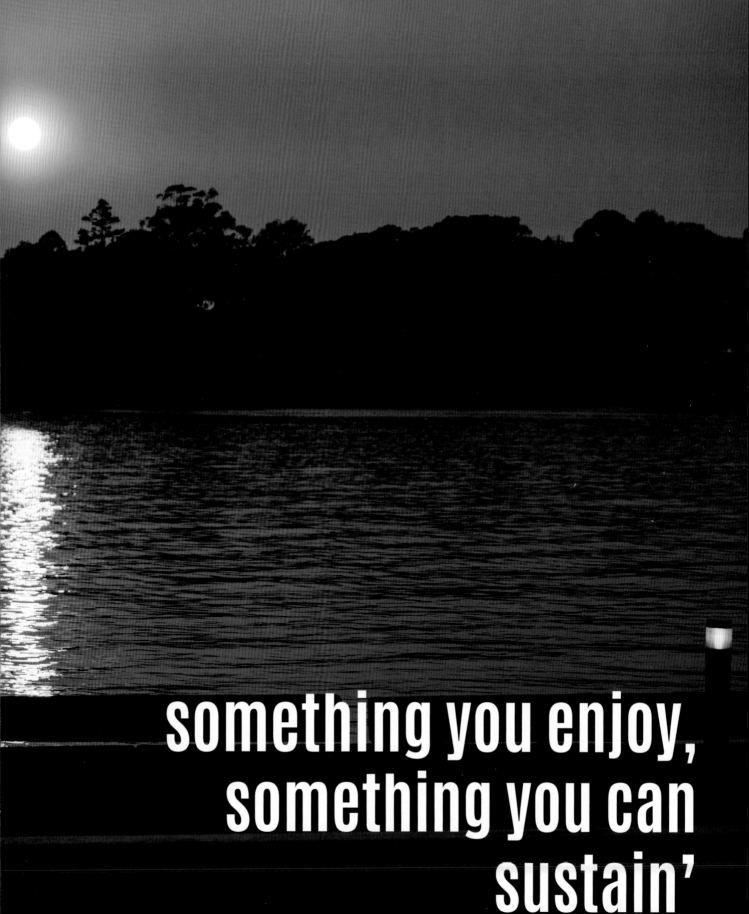

something you enjoy, something you can sustain'

DESSERT

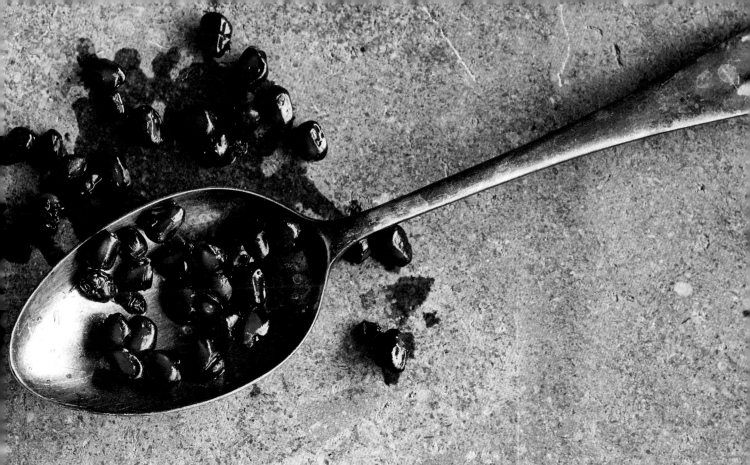

Satisfy your sweet tooth with these simple desserts that are guaranteed to put a smile on your face. Just the trick for that evening treat or weekend indulgence. Find a happy corner and just forget about the world for a moment!

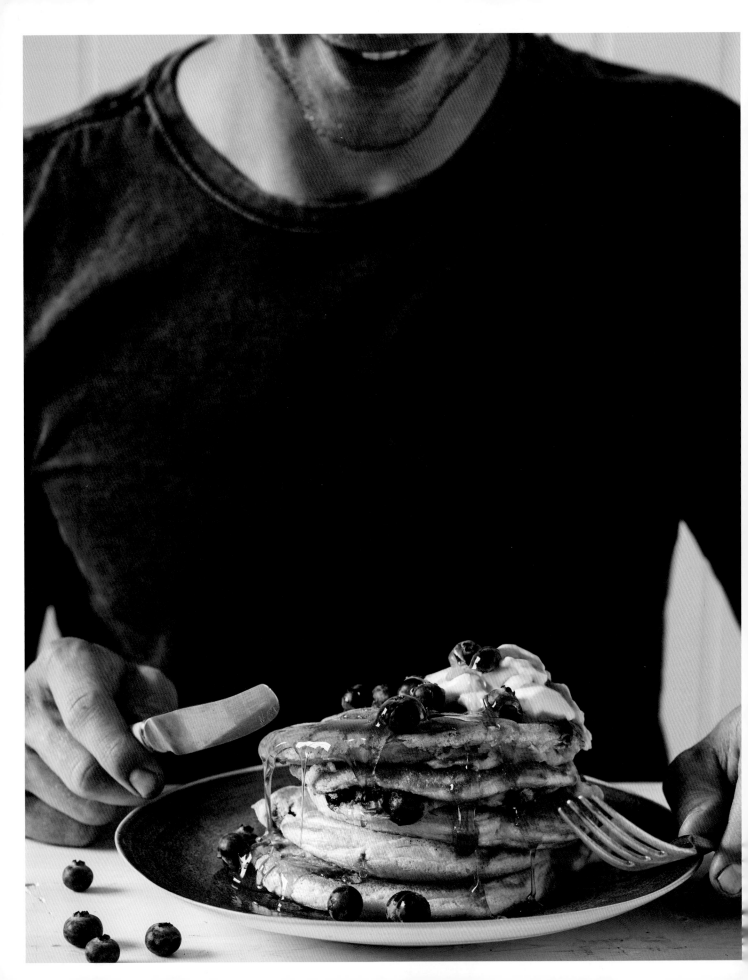

Fluffy Coconut and Blueberry Hotcakes

MAKES 6 HOTCAKES (SERVES 2)

Super light and delicious these little hotcakes are bursting with protein, making them just the perfect choice before a busy day ahead.

You will need:

½ cup plain flour

½ tsp baking powder

2 large eggs

½ cup milk

½ cup pasteurized egg whites

2 cups frozen blueberries

2 tbs coconut yoghurt

1 tbs honey

2 tbs extra virgin olive oil

salt

Simple steps:

In a large mixing bowl sift and combine the flour, baking powder and a pinch of salt. Add the whole eggs and about half the milk and start whisking, add a little more milk until you have a thick batter. In a separate bowl whisk the egg whites until light and fluffy and roughly tripled in size. Carefully fold the egg whites into the batter without losing too many of the air bubbles. Adjust the consistency by adding a little more milk if you think it needs it.

Heat a small non-stick pan over medium heat and drizzle a small amount of olive oil into the pan. Ladle a serving of batter into the pan and scatter a few frozen blueberries over the top. Drizzle a little more batter over the top, sealing the blueberries in. After about 2 minutes carefully flip the hotcake over and cook for another minute. Heat the remaining blueberries in the microwave for 1 minute then spoon over the top and serve with coconut yogurt and extra honey.

TOP TIP:

Prep ahead and make a large batch. These hotcakes freeze really well. Once cool simply wrap individually in cling film and freeze. To reheat microwave in the clingfilm and serve with warm blueberries.

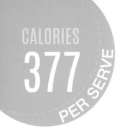
Rich Chocolate and Avocado Mousse

(SERVES 2)

Creamy and unbelievably moreish, avocado and chocolate are the perfect match.
This is everything you want from a chocolate dessert.

You will need:

1 large avocado

3 heaped tsp cacao powder

2 tsp honey

1 tsp vanilla essence

50 g (1.7 oz) 70% dark chocolate

pinch of sea salt

Simple steps:

Slice the avocado in half and remove the stone. Add the flesh to a food processor along with the cacao powder, honey, vanilla essence and a pinch of sea salt. Blend until smooth.

Serve in a bowl and grate the dark chocolate over the top.

TOP TIP:

Works really well with mixed berries or sliced banana. Ensure you cover with cling film and store in the fridge. Best enjoyed on the day of making but will happily keep for one day afterwards.

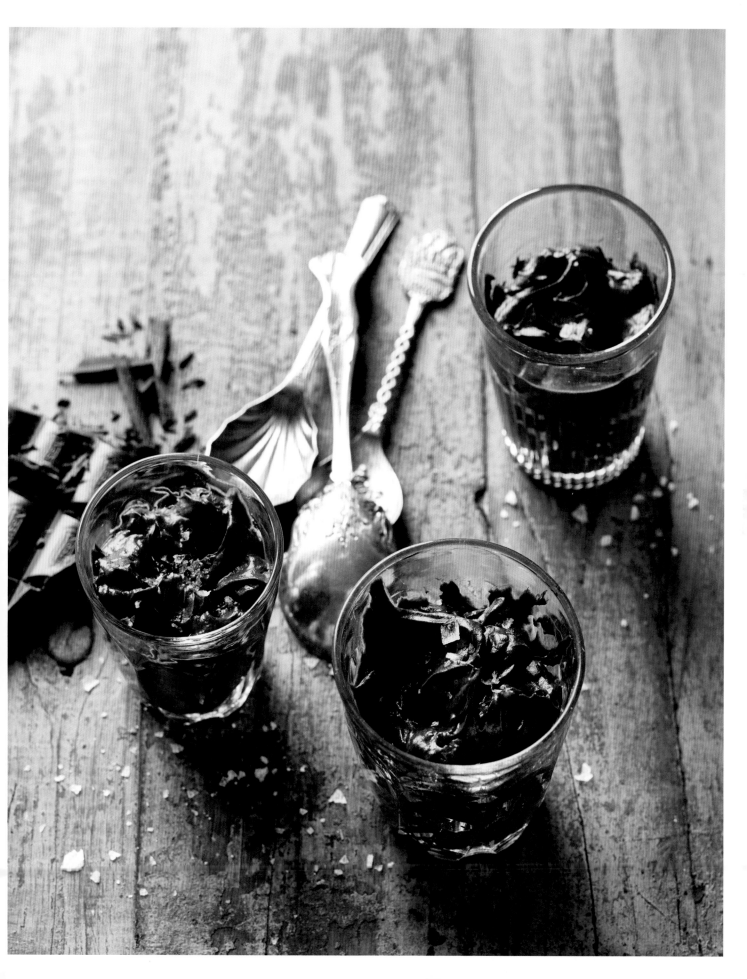

Spiced Apple and Berry Jars

(SERVES 4)

Every time I eat spiced apples and berries I think of winter, but these little jars of pure pleasure can be eaten all year round. Serve them up hot when the weather turns cold or straight from the fridge when it starts to warm up. Either way I know you'll love them!

You will need:

2 apples, diced

2 cups frozen mixed berries

1 lemon, zested and juiced

2 tsp cinnamon

1 tsp cornflour

3 tbs honey

4 tbs Greek yoghurt

Simple steps:

Place the apples and mixed berries in a pan over a low heat. Add the zest and juice from the lemon, and the cinnamon, and stir.

Mix the cornflour and a dash of water in a small bowl then add to the fruit. Once the fruit starts to soften add the honey then remove from the heat. Place a lid on for 5 minutes allowing the fruit to stew and soften a little then serve with a spoon of Greek yoghurt.

TOP TIP:

Store in individual jars in the fridge. These little fruit jars are delicious when served with Mum's 'Too Good' toasted granola (see page 41).

Banana and Blueberry Ice Cream

(SERVES 4)

There's something super satisfying about creating your own ice cream using
just a handful of ingredients.
This is the guilt-free dessert you can top with pretty much anything.

You will need:

- 4–6 medium bananas, frozen
- 1 punnet blueberries
- 3 handfuls almonds (topping)

Simple steps:

Peel the bananas and slice into quarters. Freeze in sandwich bags over night. Next day, place in a food processor or blender and blend. The consistency will change as the banana starts to soften. It will eventually become nice and creamy so stick with it and keep blending. You will have to keep stopping the blender and scrapping the banana into the middle of the blender to ensure there is enough mixture in contact with the blades.

Once soft, scrape into a bowl and either serve straight away with fresh blueberries and almonds or place into a glass bowl and refreeze. I'd recommend removing it from the freezer 10–15 minutes before you plan on enjoying it.

TOP TIP:

Try folding some cacao powder into the bananas when blending to give you a lovely chocolatey combo.

GOOD TO KNOW:

Bananas are the ultimate **quick energy source,** containing lots of natural sugars, which also make them a great dessert choice. They also contain a good amount of **potassium** and **vitamin C.**

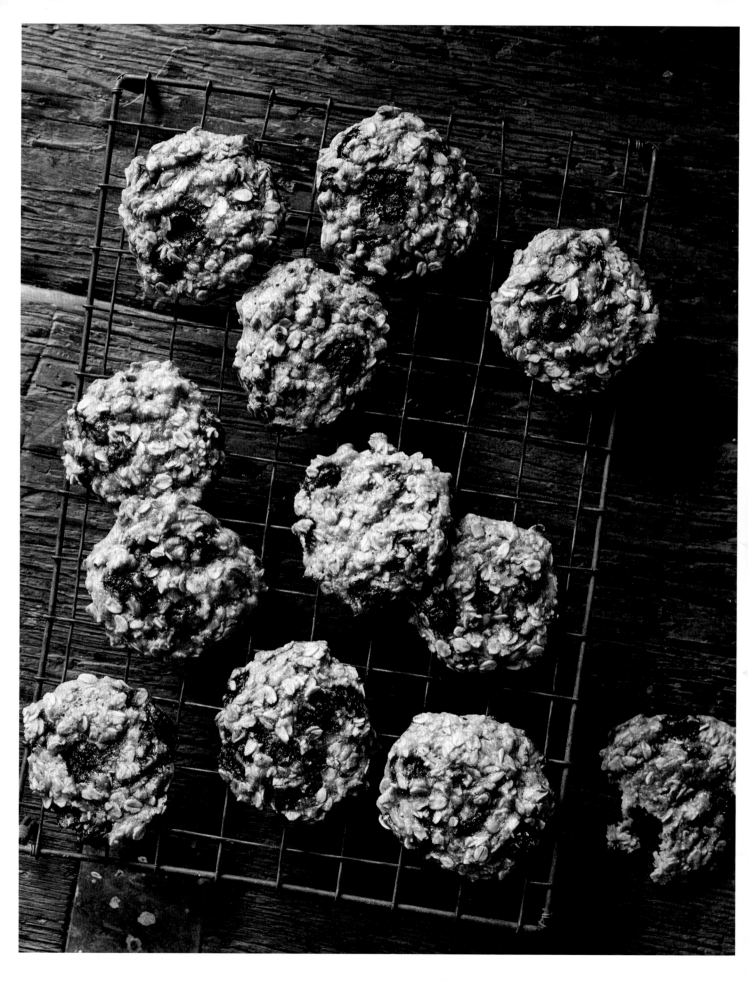

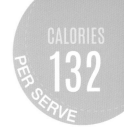
Chewy Peanut Butter and Raspberry Cookies

(MAKES 12 COOKIES)

If you can stop at just one of these yummy cookies you've got more willpower than me.
Soft, chewy, sweet and totally delicious you'll be addicted in no time. Sorry!

You will need:

- 3 ripe bananas, mashed
- 1 ½ cups porridge oats
- ½ tsp baking powder
- 1 tbsp honey
- 3 tbsp peanut butter (low sugar, low salt)
- 1 medium egg, beaten
- 1 ½ cups frozen raspberries

Simple steps:

Preheat the oven to 180°C (350°F). Mash the bananas together in a mixing bowl with a fork until they resemble a thick puree. Add the oats, baking powder, honey and peanut butter and mix well. Beat the egg separately in a small bowl then add to the oats, and finally fold in the frozen raspberries.

Line a baking tray with some greaseproof paper. Using a tablespoon, spoon a little mixture onto the tray and spread out to a cookie shape. Leave a little space around each cookie.

Bake in the oven for 18–20 minutes. Once cooked leave to cool on a wire rack.

TOP TIP:

Store in an airtight container in a cool dry place. Fancy an ice-cream sandwich? Scoop some banana and blueberry ice cream (page [XXX]) onto your cookies for the ultimate treat.

GOOD TO KNOW:

You'll have to double up on this recipe because I'm telling you now these cookies won't last.

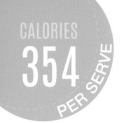

Honey and Rosemary Roast Pears

(SERVES 2)

Sweet roast pears make for a really healthy dessert that can be enjoyed any time of the day.

You will need:

- 2 ripe pears
- 1 lemon, ½ sliced, ½ juiced
- 3 tbs honey
- 1 handful walnuts, roughly chopped
- 2–3 sprigs of rosemary, roughly chopped
- 4 tbs yoghurt
- 1 tsp cinnamon
- 1 tsp vanilla essence

Simple steps:

Preheat the oven to 200°C (390°F). Slice the bottom and the top off the pears then slice in half and carefully hollow out the core, creating a small well in each half. Slice a very small piece off the skin side of the pear, allowing it to lie flat on the oven tray.

Line an oven tray with some greaseproof paper then lie the pears on the tray along with a few slices of lemon on top. Drizzle two tablespoons of honey over the top along with some lemon juice, then roast the pears in the oven for 5 minutes. Turn the pears over after 5 minutes and scatter the rosemary sprigs and chopped nuts over the pears then return to the oven for a further 5 minutes.

While the pears are roasting put the yoghurt in a small bowl, add the cinnamon, and vanilla essence, and a spoon of honey and mix well. Once the pears are cooked serve a spoon of sweetened cinnamon yoghurt in the small well of each pear and top with toasted walnuts.

TOP TIP:

Roasted pears are delicious eaten as a dessert or even chopped up and served with breakfast granola the following morning.

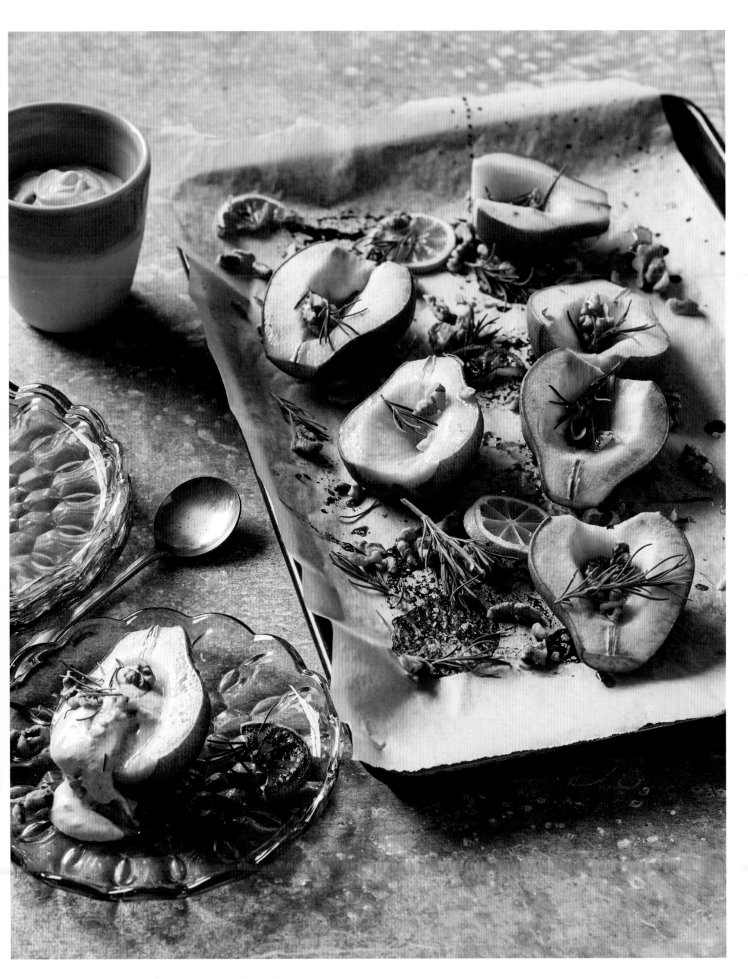

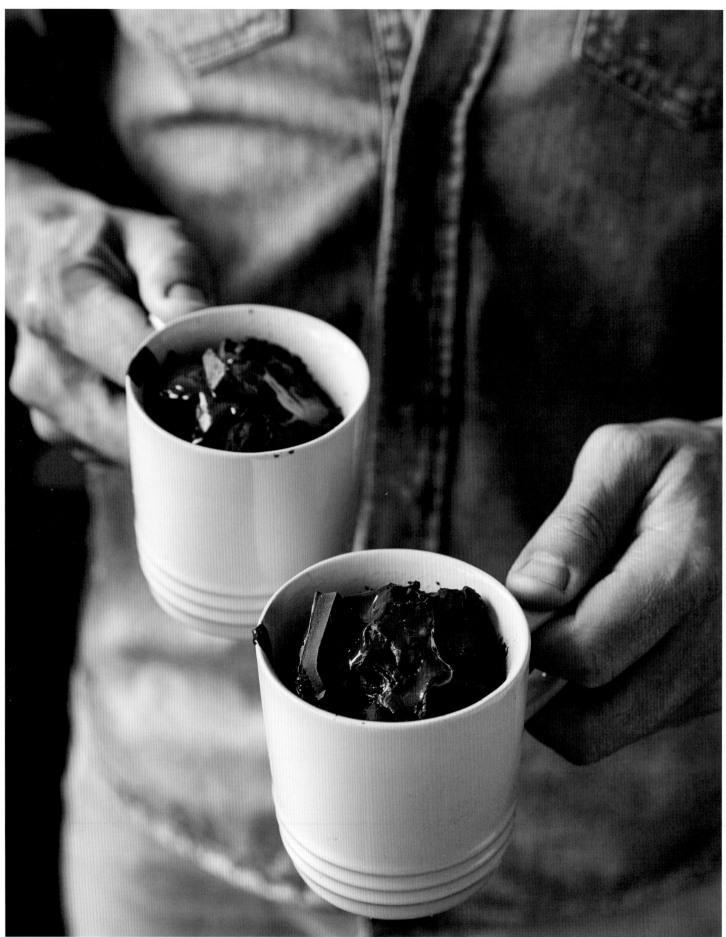

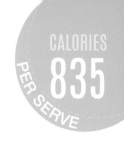

Dirty Dark Chocolate Mug Cake

(SERVES 2)

Yes, you read that right, and no your eyes are not deceiving you – that is a chocolate cake in a mug.
Oh, and by the way, it's cooked in the microwave.
One last thing, it takes less than 5 minutes from scratch.
Now do I have your attention?!

You will need:

- cup plain flour
- cup cacao powder
- 2 tbsp honey
- 4 tbsp coconut oil (solid state)
- 1 whole egg
- cup unsweetened almond milk
- 40 g (1.4 oz) 70% dark chocolate, broken into pieces

Simple steps:

Place the flour, cacao powder and honey in a bowl and mix well. Melt the coconut oil in the microwave for 45 seconds then add to the flour and mix once more.

Whisk the egg in a small bowl. Add to the mixture along with the almond milk and whisk well. Roughly chop the chocolate into small pieces and add to the mix, giving it one final whisk.

Use your fingers to rub a small amount of coconut oil into two mugs, making sure you rub it right around the base and sides. Spoon the mixture evenly into the two mugs then place in the microwave and cook on full power for 1 minute. Open the door and wait for 10–15 seconds then close the door and cook again for 15 seconds. Open the door one final time for 15 seconds then cook one final time for 15 seconds. You are heating it this way to ensure the cake doesn't explode and to keep it moist.

Be careful as the middle of the cake will be extremely hot.

TOP TIP:

You can fill the mugs with the chocolate mix then cover and store in the fridge ready to cook in under 3 minutes.

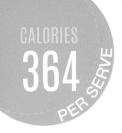

Honey-Fired Cashews

(SERVES 4)

Without a doubt the cashew is my favorite nut, and this recipe takes them from good
to unbelievable with its sweet but spicy coating. You can enjoy these honey-fired cashews
as a snack, or once cooled break them up and sprinkle them over ice cream,
some fresh fruit, or they even work over salads. Sweet as a nut!

You will need:

- 25 g (1 oz) butter
- 2 tbs honey
- ½ tsp chilli powder
- 180 g (6 oz) cashews
- 2 tbs sesame seeds
- pinch sea salt
- ½ tsp chilli flakes

Simple steps:

Preheat the oven to 180°C (350°F). Gently melt the butter, honey and chilli powder in a pan over a medium heat and stir. Line an oven tray with some greaseproof paper and scatter the nuts onto the tray. Pour the honey butter over the top. Using a spoon toss them around ensuring all the nuts are well coated. Roast in the oven for about 8 minutes, then remove and add the sesame seeds. Toss well once more with a spoon so they roast evenly and return to the oven for a final 8 minutes.

I like to finish mine with a little extra honey, some chilli flakes and a pinch of sea salt. Leave to cool then get stuck in. After about 30 minutes the nuts will stick together completely so you can then break into larger pieces.

TOP TIP:

Once cool, store in an airtight container in a cool dry place. They will also freeze really well.

GOOD TO KNOW:

These spicy cashews are a great source of **healthy fat** and a nice alternative to almonds or walnuts.

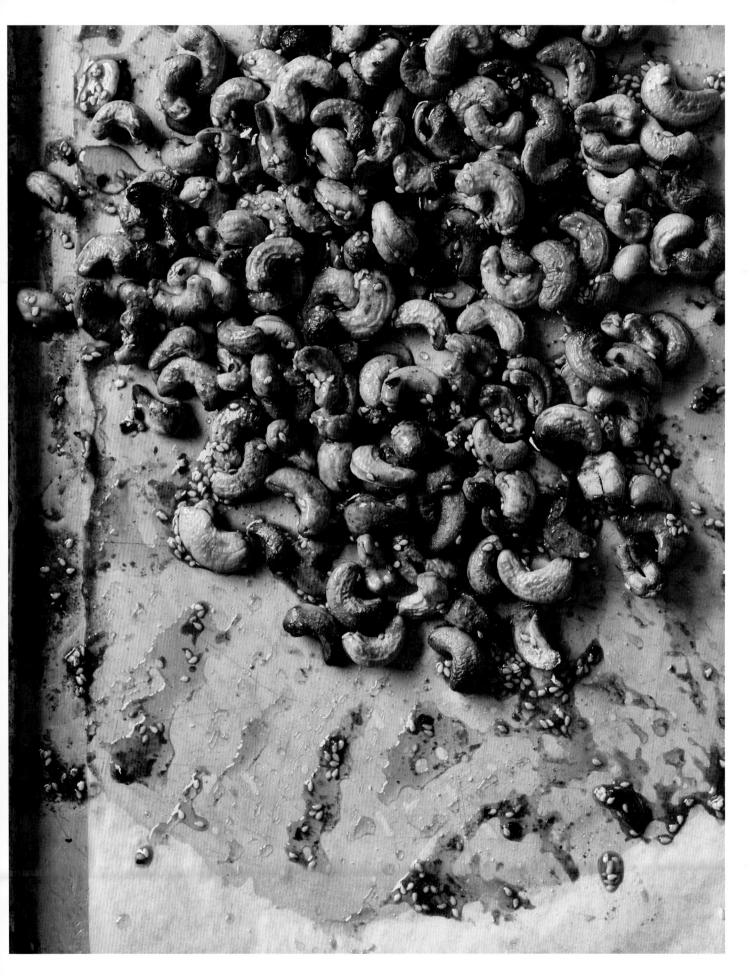

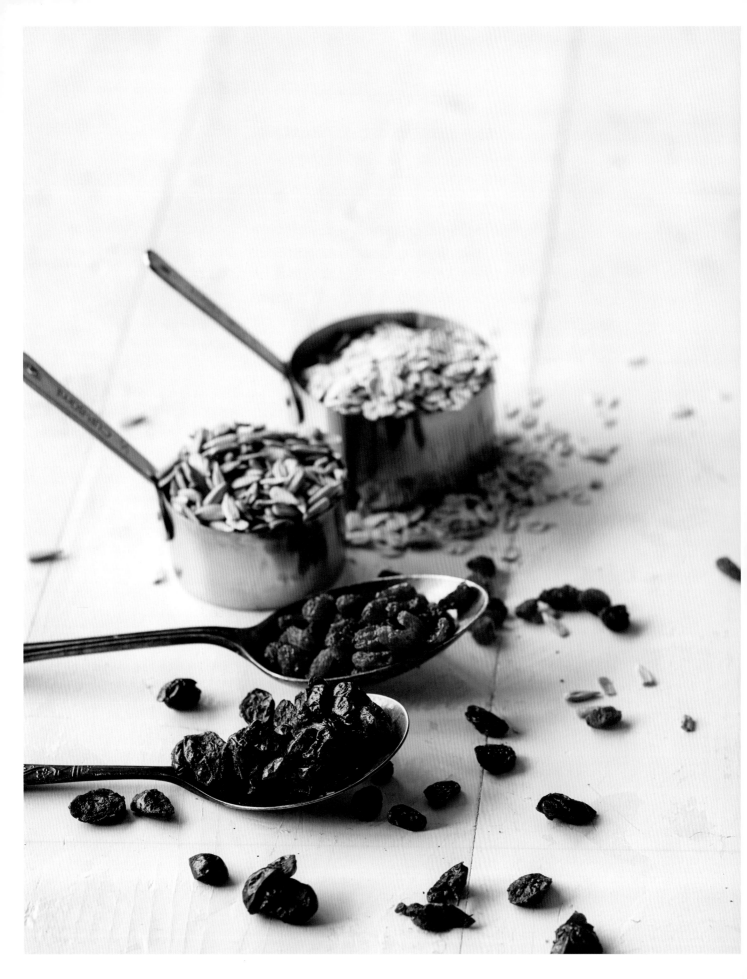

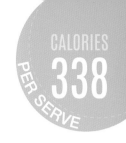

Orange, Cranberry and Pecan Energy Bars

(MAKES 12 BARS)

I love making a large batch of these bite-size bars, perfect to pop into your bag
and enjoy when you're looking for that little pick-me-up later in the day.
Just one bar provides enough energy to get you back on course.

You will need:

- 2 cups porridge oats
- 2 tsp cinnamon
- ½ cup coconut oil (solid state)
- 1 cup dried cranberries
- ½ cup nut butter
- 1 large orange, zested and juiced
- 1 cup pecans, roughly chopped

Simple steps:

Preheat the oven to 200°C (390°F). Scatter the oats and cinnamon onto an ovenproof tray lined with baking paper. Roast in the oven for 10 minutes.

Melt the coconut oil in a microwave for 45 seconds then transfer to a food processor with the cranberries, nut butter, orange zest and half the juice and blend. You can also do this by hand if you wish, just make sure you mix the ingredients together well.

Place the toasted oats in a mixing bowl and fold in the cranberry mix along with the chopped pecans. Slice the skin off the other half of the orange and roughly chop the flesh into small pieces, then add to the oats and mix well. Ensure there are no pips in the orange before you begin slicing it up.

Mix all the ingredients together then line a 20 x 20 cm (8 x 8 in) tin with greaseproof paper and press the mix into the tin. Place the tin in the freezer for 20 minutes until set, then you can slice into individual bars and store in the fridge in an airtight container.

TOP TIP:

Once the bars have been sliced, wrap each bar individually and store in the freezer to extend the shelf life. Remove 20 minutes before you are ready to enjoy.

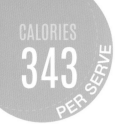

Perfect Popcorn - Three Ways

(SERVES 3)

Look like a boss in the kitchen by creating the most amazing homemade popcorn.
The best part about this is it's super fun. Right before your eyes the kernels
will burst into life leaving you with the most amazingly crunchy, delicious popcorn,
perfect for a cozy night in.

You will need:

4–6 tbs sunflower oil

100 g (3.5 oz) popcorn kernels

25 g unsalted butter

3 tbs honey

generous pinch of sea salt

½ tsp paprika

Simple steps:

Place the oil in a large, thick-bottomed pan over a medium-to-high heat for 1–2 minutes. Add 1–2 kernels to see if the oil is hot enough – you'll know if it is because they will quickly transform into popcorn. Once hot enough, tip the rest of the kernels into the pan and place a lid on. Continue to shake the pan as this will cover the kernels in the hot oil and start the cooking process. After about 30–45 seconds remove the pan from the heat but keep shaking until you hear the popping stop. If you don't hear too much popping return the pan to the heat and repeat that step. Once ready tip the popcorn onto a large tray then separate into three serving bowls.

Honey butter: Melt the butter in a small pan and add the honey, stirring well. Once mixed pour over the top of one of the bowls of popcorn and mix well.

Salted: Sprinkle a generous pinch of salt over the second bowl.

Paprika: Add a dusting of paprika and salt over the third bowl.

TOP TIP:

Once cool, store in an airtight container for a winning mid-morning snack. The popcorn will stay crunchy for at least two days.

GOOD TO KNOW:

Popcorn can actually be a great **low-calorie** snack when you serve it plain and with just a pinch of salt.

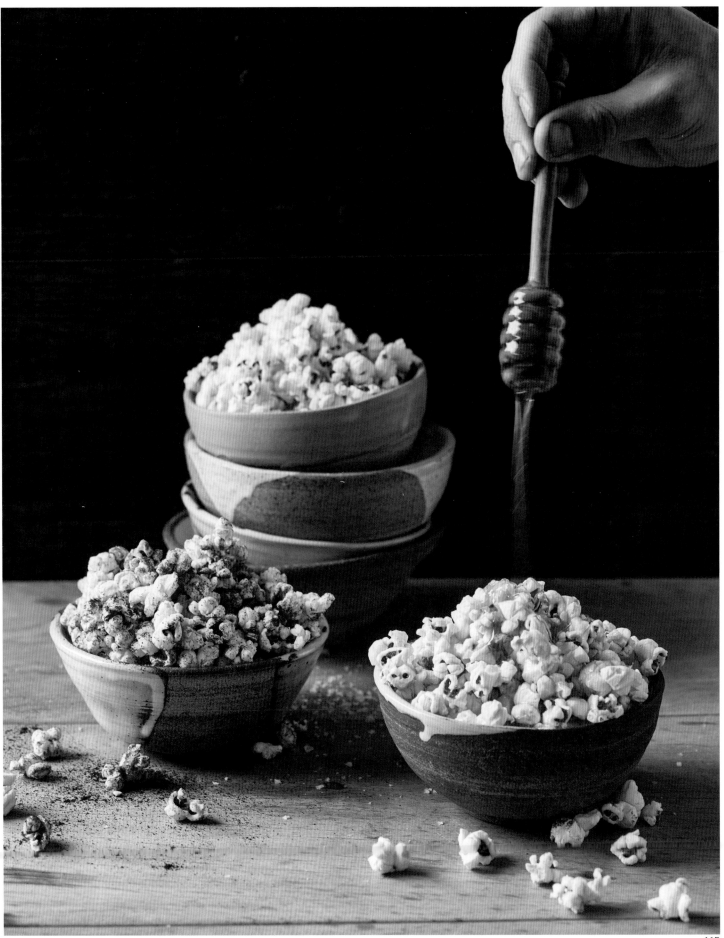

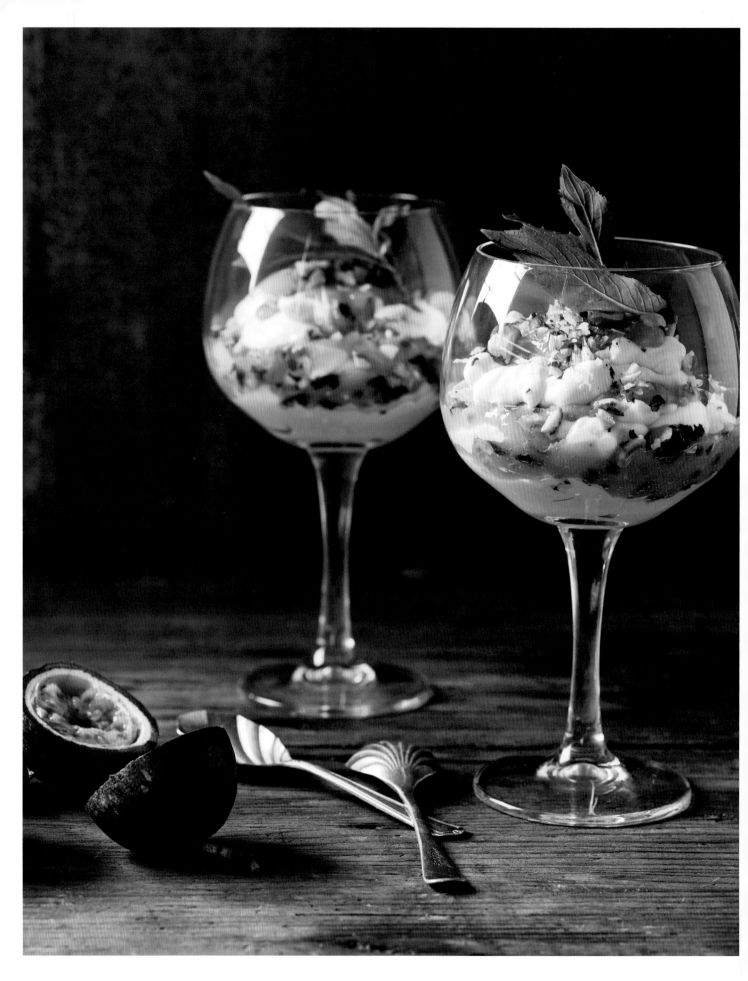

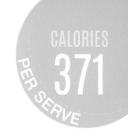

Mango and Passionfruit Trifle

(SERVES 2)

I'm not really sure if this sits in the dessert or breakfast section.
I know one thing for sure though, whatever time you choose to eat this you're going to
absolutely love it. Juicy mango and passionfruit puree layered between coconut yoghurt
is just the beginning; throw in some toasted hazelnuts and this is one stunning dessert.

You will need:

- 2 handfuls hazelnuts, crushed
- 2 tsp honey
- 1 mango, diced
- 4 passionfruit
- 1 lime, zested
- 6 tbs coconut yoghurt

Simple steps:

Preheat the oven to 180°C (350°F). Scatter the hazelnuts onto an oven tray lined with greaseproof paper and drizzle with honey. Roast in the oven for 8–10 minutes then remove and allow to cool.

Remove the flesh from the mango and place in a food processor. Blend for 20–30 seconds until smooth then spoon into a bowl. Slice the passion fruit in half and scoop the seeds straight into the mango puree and mix well.

In a separate bowl, add the lime zest to the yoghurt and mix well. Spoon about a tablespoon of yoghurt into the bottom of a glass, then add the mango and passion fruit puree. Once the nuts have cooled, roughly chop and add a small handful. Repeat this process until you have used all the ingredients, aiming to finish the layers with puree then nuts on top.

TOP TIP:

Cover and store in the fridge for 2–3 days. Roast some extra hazelnuts and once cooled store these in an airtight container. Hazelnuts are great crumbled over the top of porridge, or a fruit salad.

GOOD TO KNOW:

Just one cup of mango hits 100% of your daily **vitamin C** needs. Good times!

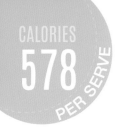

Salted Chocolate and Coconut Cake

(SERVES 8)

So technically this isn't a 20-minute recipe. I mean it takes 20 minutes to make but it needs
a little time to set (1–2 hours) but trust me it will be totally worth it,
because you'll be left with a naughty little chocolate coconut cake that's simply to die for.

You will need:

1 ½ cups porridge oats

¼ cup pistachios

¼ cup cashews

5 tbs coconut oil (solid state)

6 tbs honey

6 leaves gelatin (10 g/0.3 oz)

400 ml (13.5 fl oz) coconut cream

200 g (7 oz) 70% dark chocolate, roughly
   chopped

½ cup coconut flakes or desiccated coconut

1 tsp sea salt

Simple steps:

Grease and line the bottom and sides of a 20 cm (8 in) round cake tin with some baking paper.

Place the oats, and nuts in a food processor and blend until you have coarse crumbs then tip into a mixing bowl. Melt the coconut oil in a microwave for 45 seconds then add to the oat mix along with 3 tablespoons of honey and mix well. Push the oat mix firmly into the bottom of the lined cake tin and place in the fridge to chill while you make the mousse.

Add the gelatin sheets to a bowl of lukewarm water for 3–5 minutes until soft.

Gently warm the coconut cream in a pan then break up 150 g of chocolate and start adding to the cream while stirring. Don't allow the cream to boil. Keep stirring until all of the chocolate has melted then add the remaining honey and a generous pinch of salt.

Once the gelatin has softened transfer to a small saucepan and gently melt over a low heat. It will only take a few seconds to melt then stir into the chocolate cream. Remove the cake tin from the fridge and pour the chocolate cream over the top of the oats. Give the dish one small tap on the bench to break any air bubbles that may have formed then sprinkle the coconut flakes over the top.

Return to the fridge for an hour or so to set. Just before you are ready to slice add an extra sprinkling of sea salt and some grated chocolate.

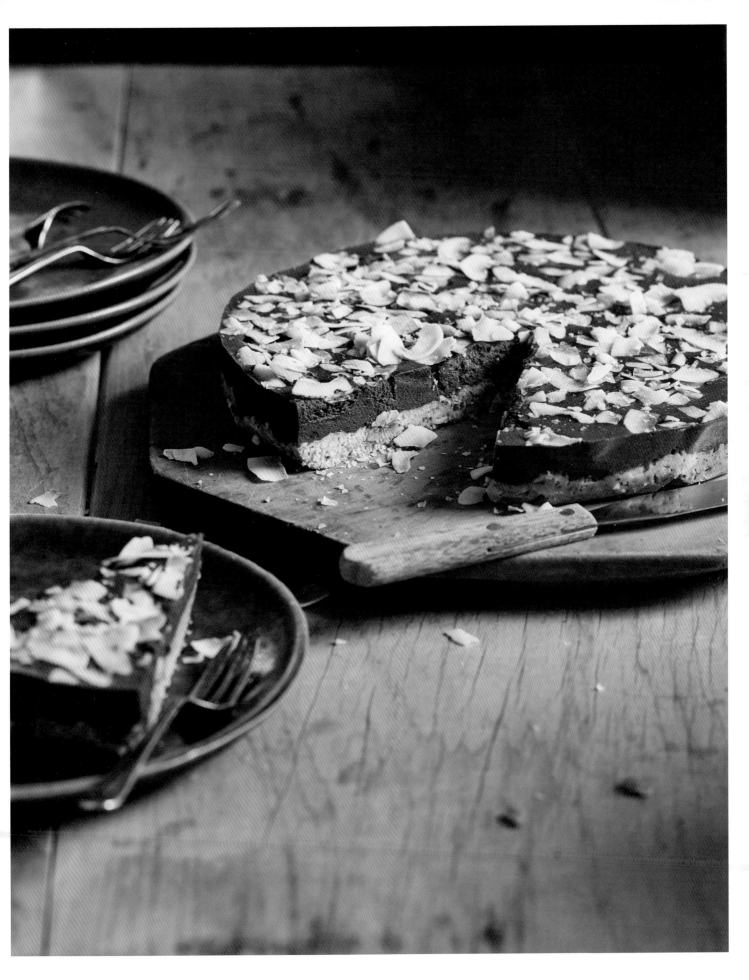

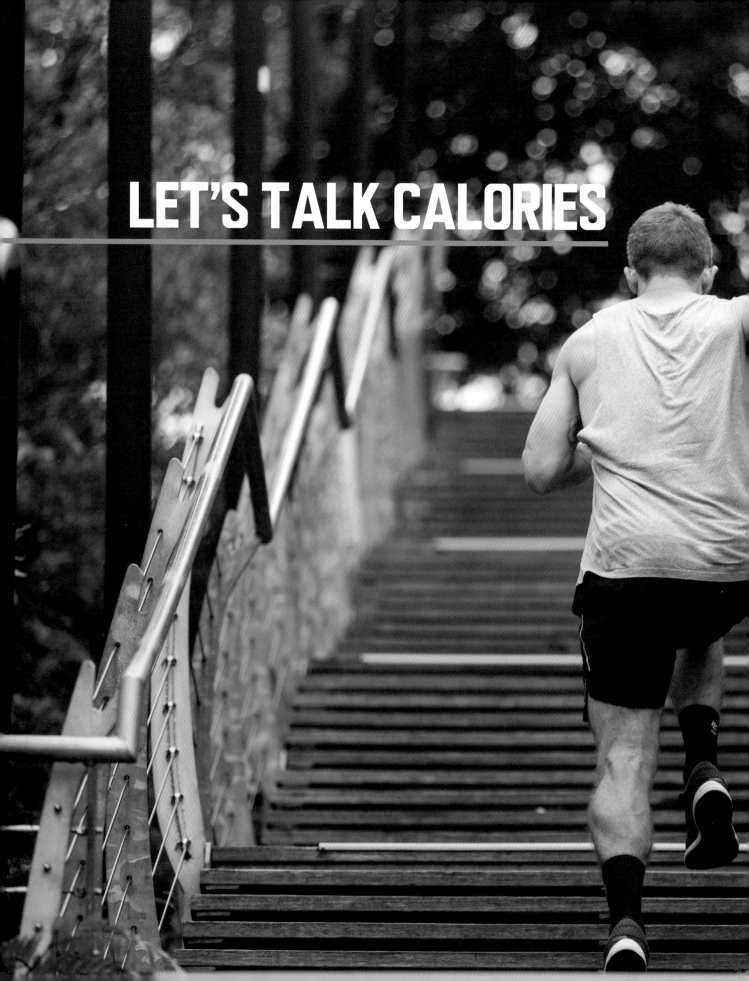

LET'S TALK CALORIES

Calories are the amount of energy in food, sometimes referred to as 'joules' but they really mean the same thing. One calorie is equal to 4.18 joules so if you consume 500 calories, you're consuming 2090 joules of energy.

That's important to know because nutritional labels on food don't always write calories next to the food item, often they will write kilojoules or kJ. It's easy to find out the calorie amount by simply dividing the kilojoule amount by 4.18.

For example, an 850 (kj) snack (850 ÷ 4.18) = 203 calories

When looking to change your body composition it's imperative you look at your nutrition first. Exercise and training are a secondary aspect and cannot outweigh (excuse the pun) a bad diet.

Calorie deficit or negative energy balance is where your body doesn't get the calories it requires to perform maintenance of your current body weight.

Calorie surplus or positive energy balance is where your body gets more calories than it requires to perform maintenance of your current body weight.

RMR or **resting metabolic rate** is the rate at which your body burns energy when it is at complete rest and just performing essential functions like breathing, circulating blood etc. Think of it like lying down on a couch and doing absolutely nothing kind of rest.

Now this is fairly useless information for 99% of us because we aren't sitting on a couch all day; we move and we exercise so we need to find out how much energy our body expends daily in order to work out how much food we need to eat to balance everything out or to create a slight deficit if weight loss is the goal.

TDEE or total daily energy expenditure is the total number of calories your body will burn in a day including physical activity such as exercise. As discussed, in order to prevent weight gain you must balance out your daily calorie intake with your daily energy expenditure so you can see why knowing these numbers will help you to understand how much you need to eat in order to hit your goal.

NEAT or non-exercise activity thermogenesis is the low intensity activities we do such as light walks, tasks around the house, moving, stretching etc. These activities although very low in terms of burning calories, when done for long enough can actually be really great for overall health and also weight loss so you can include this as a contributor to affecting your metabolism.

Did you know? It takes about 3500 calories to burn 1 pound (0.5 kg) of fat. Now this seems like a lot of work and I'm not saying you need to burn all 3500 calories through exercise, no, there is a much simpler and easier way to do it. By reducing your daily intake by 500 calories over a seven-day period you will be burning up to 3500 calories (500 x 7). This is the best way to tackle weight loss, little by little and over time for long-term results.

Want To Lose Fat?

It's about getting your nutrition right. Want to put on weight? Yep you guessed it, it's about getting your nutrition right. Keep it simple though, don't try and change too much too quickly.

Why Do So Many People Fail?

Often, it's because they choose a diet they just can't sustain. The diet is either way too restrictive, and once they have finished, they put all the weight back on again or they try to change too much too quickly and don't even make it to the end, falling off track after only a few weeks in.

They may then start again a few months later and go back and forth like this, which is called yo-yo dieting. The issue with yo-yo dieting is that every time you start afresh it gets harder and harder because you can tend to lose confidence and struggle to build up the motivation to give it another go.

Calorie Cycling for Fat Loss

Our lives are busy and one day is usually different to the next. We may have work lunches, dinners out or indulgent weekends to contend with, making it difficult to follow a strict routine. Calorie cycling can be a really great way to ensure you don't plateau with your weight loss and instead continue to make progress with your fat-loss journey. It's also a great way to maintain the weight you've lost without yo-yoing back and forth.

Now obviously you need to ensure you're in, yes, you guessed it, a **_calorie deficit_** overall, but the way to effectively calorie cycle is to include higher calorie days and lower calorie days throughout your week. As long as on average and at the end of the week you are in a deficit, it will work.

As an example, let's say we take 2500 calories as your suggested daily calorie intake. For weight maintenance. Our first step as you know is to reduce those calories by 500 (see page 13 for simple weight loss tips reminder) from there all you need to do is to choose four lower calorie days and three higher calorie days, which could look like this:'

Monday: 2200

Tuesday: 2000

Wednesday: 2200

Thursday: 2000

Friday: 2200

Saturday: 2000

Sunday: 2200

Let's do some quick maths and see how this works:

2200 x 4 (Mon, Wed, Fri, Sun) + 2000 x 3 (Tue, Thu, Sat) = 14,800 ÷ 7 (days) = 2114 calories

Remember, as long as you are under your suggested calorie intake as an average for the entire week then you are on the right track.

I would suggest you stick to the lower calorie days when you are not exercising and then higher calorie days when you have exercise sessions planned, as you will need the extra fuel to get you through the session and to help with recovery.

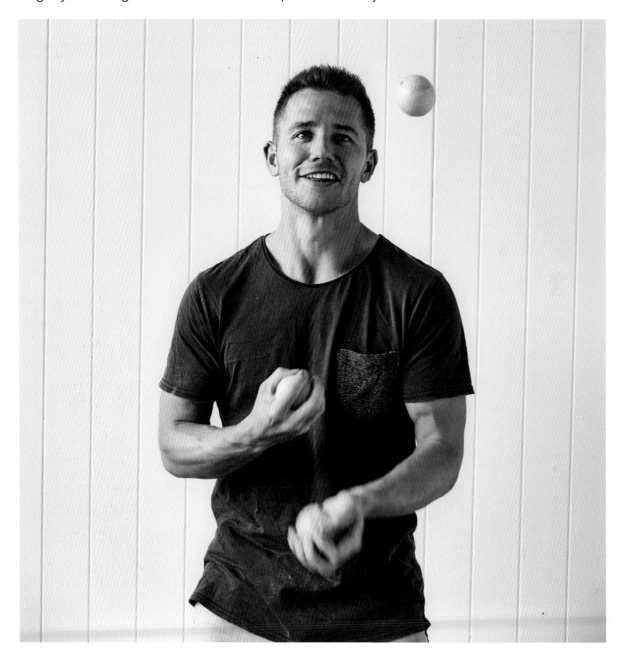

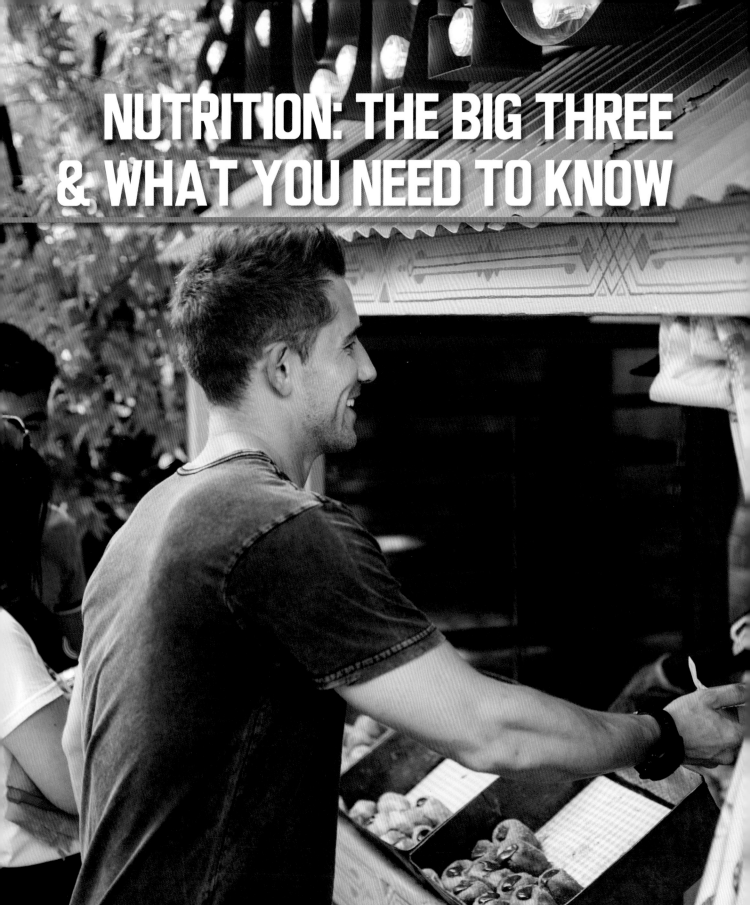

NUTRITION: THE BIG THREE & WHAT YOU NEED TO KNOW

Proteins, fats and carbohydrates are essential to keeping us alive, maintaining or changing our body composition and most importantly recovering effectively from exercise. These macronutrients provide the body with the energy it needs in order to function efficiently.

Everyone Loves Carbohydrates

Carbohydrates are often labelled as the 'bad guys' of food and a lot of people avoid them thinking it will help to lose weight. However, we need to get away from thinking carbohydrates are bad.

Carbohydrates are essential in our diet as they provide our body with valuable energy. There are lots of healthy carbs out there and they can be found in unprocessed whole grains, vegetables, salads and fruit. The more 'unhealthy' forms are found in white bread, pastries and highly processed or refined foods.

When we perform intense exercise, we will use carbohydrates as our main energy source, which is why we must make sure we have adequate stores in our body. In order to tap into this energy our body must first break down the dietary carbohydrates we consume, extracting the glucose. Once the glucose has been absorbed into the body some travels off to the blood and the brain and the rest travels to the liver and the muscles to be stored as glycogen. It remains there until we need it again for energy but must be converted back into glucose first before we can use it. Incorporating a good mixture of whole grain carbohydrates into our diet is the key to long term health.

Packed with Protein

Perhaps one of the most important micro nutrients that is often overlooked is protein. Along with regulating our metabolism and producing hormones, protein provides us with the fuel our body and muscles need in order to function and grow. Protein is made up of amino acids – think of these like the building blocks that give protein its structure. There are two types of amino acids, non-essential and essential. The body has the ability to make non-essential amino acids, but it cannot make essential amino acids; as a result we need to get these from our diet. An added bonus is that a high protein diet, when consumed with carbohydrates, will leave you feeling fuller for longer.

The Right Fat

Fat contains a lot more calories per gram than carbohydrate and protein, therefore we don't need to consume as much. This also means that it is easy to overeat fat, and even though some fats may be deemed as 'good fats', consuming too much of anything can lead to weight gain. Dietary fat, or fat that is found naturally in our foods has several roles; along with providing an energy source to the body, it also transports certain vitamins effectively throughout the body.

Types of Fat

Saturated fat is easy to consume in large amounts but very stubborn to shift when it comes to exercise, so be mindful of how much you are eating. Saturated fats include:

- meat
- butter
- cheese
- cream

Unsaturated fat is split into two categories, monounsaturated and polyunsaturated. Both can help you improve your heart health. These healthy fats help our body metabolize efficiently and absorb nutrients properly.

Monounsaturated fats include:

- olive oil
- avocado
- peanuts
- almonds

Polyunsaturated fats include:

- omega 3 and 6 found in fish and chia seeds
- flax seeds and oil
- hemp
- canola oil

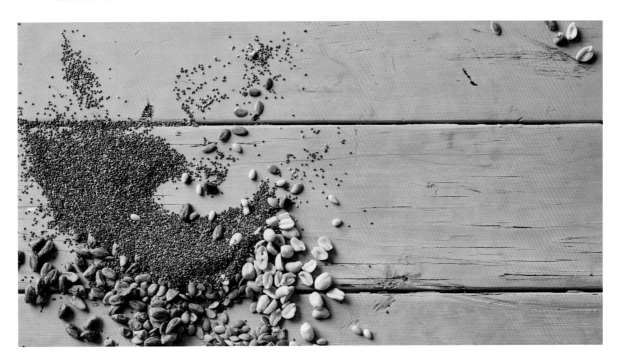

The Right Fuel to Suit Your Body Type

Finding out what body type you are can help guide you on what type of foods to eat, what foods your body deals with best and which foods to include or avoid in order to perform at your best. Body shapes are generally broken down into three types:

1 ECTOMORPH

Typical body shape being long and thin, generally quite slim with low body fat. **Ectomorphs deal with carbohydrates well. You should include these after exercise and with each meal.**

2 MESOMORPH

Has a solid frame, slight v-shaped body, with a small waist and athletic build. **Moderate tolerance to carbohydrates, so aim to eat these first thing in the morning and after exercise for best results.**

3 ENDOMORPH

Tend to have wider, pear-shaped hips and stores fat fairly easily. **Endomorphs generally don't deal with lots of carbohydrates well. Try to include carbohydrates, mainly after you have exercised. Focus on large amounts of colourful and green leafy vegetables and lean protein.**

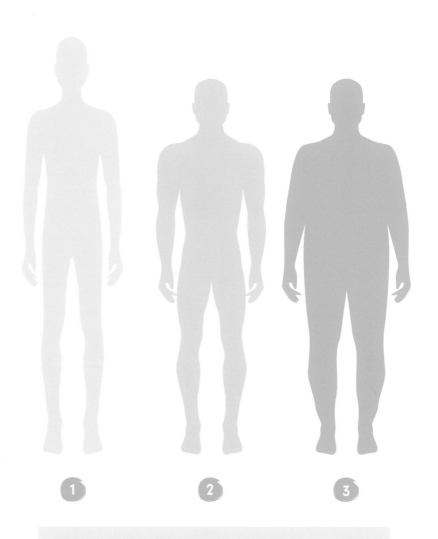

If you are unsure which body type you fall into, or you think you may be a cross between two body types (which is fairly common) and your goal is fat loss/weight loss, start by following the **endomorph** guidelines.

FOOD HACKS TO STAY AHEAD OF THE GAME!

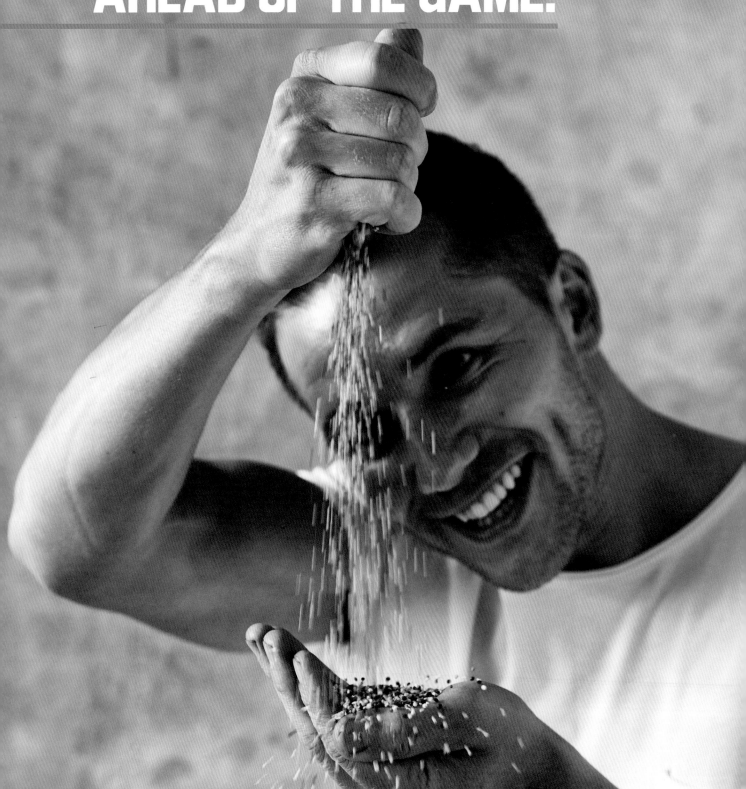

Even though all of the recipes in this book only take **20 minutes** or less to knock up, I want to make your life even easier by showing you how preparing food in advance can save you even more time in the long run.

Prepping ahead doesn't have to mean making a week's worth of food in one go and spending hours in the kitchen over the weekend. No! It can be as simple as doubling up on recipes you like or cooking a few extra pieces of meat or fish, portions of rice or extra roasted veggies, ready to add to a salad when you are on the run and only have a few minutes to spare.

I want you to enjoy cooking, and not feel like it's a chore getting the pots and pans out. A healthy relationship with food is essential to long-term health, and any quick wins along the way can make a huge difference.

Quick ingredient wins include using:

- Instant microwaveable rice and quinoa
- Tinned lentils and chicken peas
- Frozen vegetables
- Pre-mixed salads and stir-frys
- Liquid vegetable or meat stocks

This is fresh food that has either been frozen or packed to make your life easier so don't be scared to use it, as it will **save you time** in the kitchen.

Cupboard Staples

Having a well-stocked cupboard makes cooking a breeze. Half of the recipes I create start with me asking myself 'Okay, what have I got in the cupboard and how can I make this taste amazing?'

Extra virgin olive oil: I use this in just about every recipe and it's great for heart health

Salt and pepper: Help to bring out the flavor in food

Fresh garlic: So universal and really makes a difference to food

Chilli flakes: Pack some instant heat

Ground cumin: Adds a wonderful depth of flavor to meat or vegetables

Mixed herbs: Great addition to chicken, pork or roasted veggies

Vegetable stock cubes or liquid stock: Creates speedy soups in minutes

Coconut oil: A great alternative to butter when baking

Peanut butter (low salt and sugar): I mean apart from tasting great straight from the jar, I'll add it to smoothies, or as a main ingredient when baking yummy desserts

Oats: These are my breakfast staple, packed full of long-lasting energy and super cheap

Vinegar: Added to a dressing it instantly turns a salad into something amazing

Fill Your Fridge

Most of us are creatures of habit and as a result pick up the same produce from the store week-in week-out. Here's what I like to have in my fridge to make sure I can knock up something super tasty and with ease.

Spinach: Great to add to a salad or breakfast smoothie

Sweet potatoes: Roasted or even microwaved I'll serve them alongside a lunchtime omelet or as part of an evening meal

Cherry tomatoes: Eaten whole or sliced through a salad they're great

Eggs: Scrambled, poached or fried, eggs are a staple I just can't live without

Cottage cheese: Wicked when spread over toast and enjoyed with smoked salmon

Broccolini: Served with a side of protein, these superfood veggies roast wonderfully with a little olive oil and salt and pepper

Almond milk: Yummy in a breakfast smoothie every single day

Natural yoghurt: Either spooned over fruit, eaten straight from the pot or used as a marinade, yoghurt is great to use in cooking

Good to Have in the Freezer

Blueberries or mixed berries: Great to throw into a breakfast smoothie and packed full of nutrients

Peas: Steam for 2 minutes and add to a lunch or dinner

Frozen bananas: Blended with peanut butter to make the most incredible ice cream or thrown into a breakfast smoothie

Edamame beans: Add to a stir-fry or soup to boost the goodness and adds a nice bit of texture

Equipment I Can't Live Without

You don't need to spend a fortune on kitchen equipment to cook yummy food but having just a few useful tools and bits of equipment really will make your time in the kitchen more enjoyable when you're whipping up a storm.

Some equipment I use on a daily basis:

Sharp knives: Quickly and easily slice and dice vegetables with precision. Spend as much money as you can afford on these; they'll last you a lifetime if you look after them

Large chopping board: Makes chopping vegetables easy without spilling onto the kitchen bench

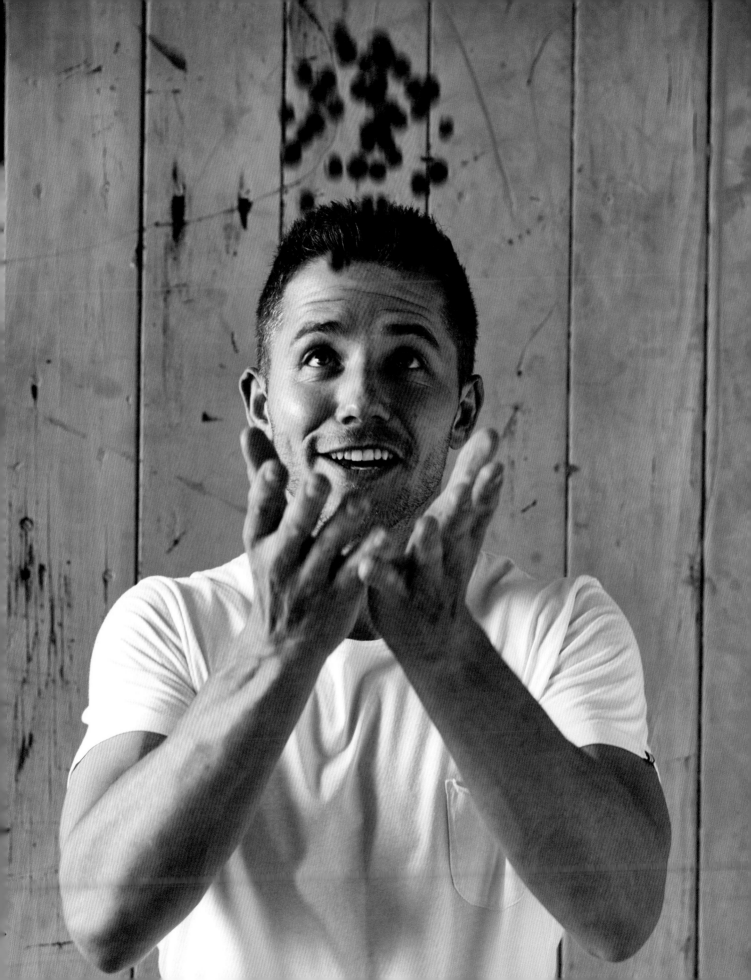

Non-stick frying pan: Use less oil when cooking and you don't have to worry about your food sticking

Set of measuring cups or spoons: Makes it easy to follow recipes accurately and hit your portion-size requirements with a set of these cups

Large mixing bowls: Whether it's mixing, marinating or stirring, the bigger the bowl, the easier you can work with the food

Selection of cooking pots: The better the quality the longer they will last

Silicon spatula: Great for stir-frys, omelets, and to scrape every last bit of ingredients from the bowl

Food processor: Optional but a nice thing to have to make chopping, blending or pulsing a breeze

Microplane or fine grater: Not very common to have in household kitchens but I'm telling you this piece of kit will help you out no end. Great for zesting citrus fruits quickly or grating whole garlic cloves.

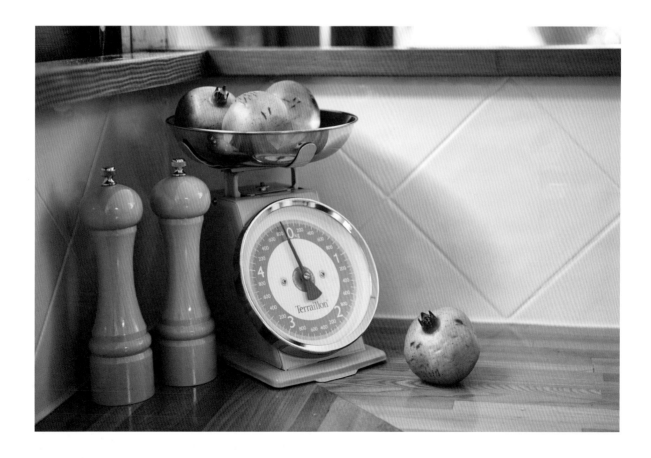

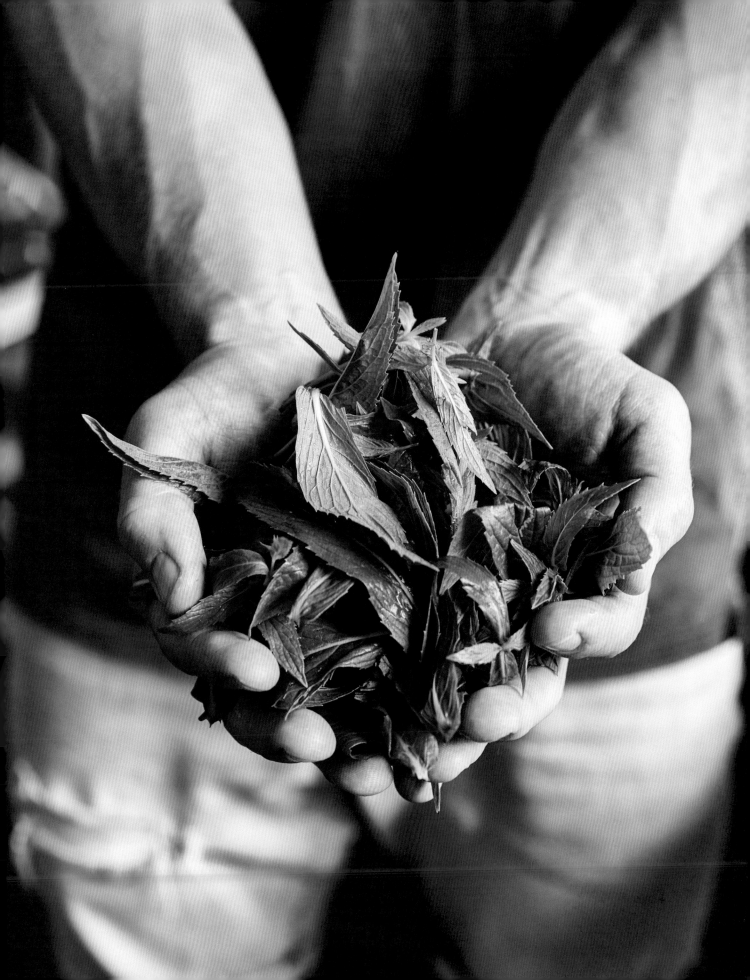

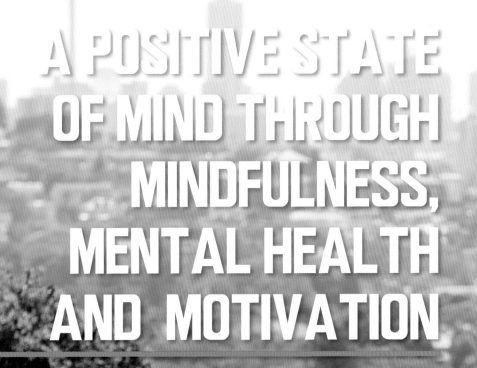

A POSITIVE STATE OF MIND THROUGH MINDFULNESS, MENTAL HEALTH AND MOTIVATION

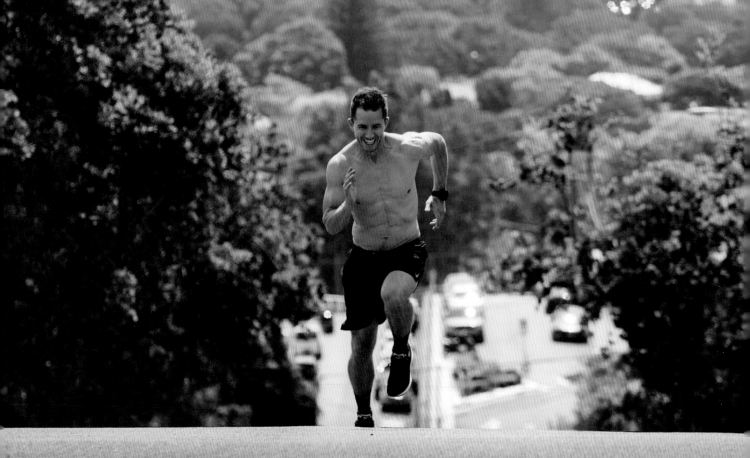

Your first stop to becoming more positive should be to check in on your physical health, because the feel-good endorphins released from exercise are incredibly powerful and the more regularly you exercise the more regular the hit of endorphins you're exposed to. If you think about it, it's also a free form of therapy that everyone has access to. So, get out there and move your body, doing something you enjoy, and you will soon start to see results. A fit body creates a fit mind and vice versa. Plus, you really can't get this part wrong; there is no right or wrong way to go about this, so don't panic. If you enjoy doing it, it gets your body moving and your mind working then it's a BIG yes from me!

But what happens if you struggle to even get motivated to start exercising? I knew that question was coming, here are my top tips to help you get off the couch and onto greatness!

Do what you enjoy: Write down five of your favorite things to do which involve you being active. Don't overthink them; if you enjoy doing them they go on the list.

Remember how you felt afterwards: Once you have finished the activity write down how you felt, as these are great to look back on the next time you're feeling demotivated and uninspired to move.

Promote healthy habits: Mark a time in your diary to do something for YOU, it could be a yoga session, a walk or a swim. The point is, if it's booked in it becomes a priority, just like any other appointment you'd make.

Get a friend on board: The next time you do any of these activities, take a friend along with you. Involving someone else will not only make it more fun but also help to keep you accountable. Celebrating success is way more fun with someone else there with you.

Mindfulness

Practicing mindfulness could be as simple as going for a walk and having a little check-in with yourself along the way. Think of it like a little service for your mind, allowing it to recharge and reset.

I'll often go for a walk and think to myself 'OK, what is going well in my life right now, what do I need to work on, what is making me happy and what is making me feel unhappy?' Then I'll try to action some of these points or share them with close friends and family. I'd encourage you to write these down as well so you can review them at a later date.

Yoga gets you double points when improving mindfulness, as it allows you to bring your mind and body together. I find a yoga session to be unlike any other form of exercise; it's almost a euphoric feeling after a class that you really can't beat. If you aren't already including yoga in your lifestyle, I would encourage you to do so.

Meditation is a great way to practice mindfulness. We live in such a busy world where things are demanded from us almost 24 hours of the day. Ever feel like you're just struggling to keep your head above water? Meditation is a great way to help reduce levels of anxiety, to connect with your surroundings and to help regulate your sleep patterns. The best news is it's free, very easy to do and in just 10 minutes it can leave you feeling incredible.

How to do it:

Get outside: Try to pick a spot out in the fresh air, ideally first thing in the morning. If you're lucky enough to do this while catching a sunrise then that's a bonus, as this will only help to bring positive vibes to the day ahead.

Get comfortable: Sit up straight, make sure you are relaxed then close your eyes and take a couple of deep breaths in and a couple of deep breaths out. Try to direct the breathing from deep within your belly.

Relax: If your mind starts to wander soon after you close your eyes don't panic, this is why you are doing it. Keep the deep breaths coming and aim to stay relaxed. You can also try box breathing to help you to stay focused and present in the moment. Breathing in only through the nose inhale for 4–5 seconds, then hold the breath for 4–5 seconds, then exhale through the nose for 4–5 seconds then hold for another 4–5 seconds, repeat these five times then go back to regular breathing.

Keep it short: Aim to sit for 5–10 minutes to begin with, then as you get more comfortable with it you can go for a little longer.

Mental health

In my experience, practicing mindfulness can also improve your mental health to help shape a more positive state of mind. I have seen firsthand through my dad what happens when you don't make your physical and mental health a priority. I would give anything to turn back the clock and get Dad exercising or enjoying a hobby, taking him away from the work environment that consumed him.

To ensure you look after your own mental health and wellbeing you must first ask yourself the question 'Are you OK?' It's basic first aid to make sure that you are OK before helping others.

Some quick wins to look after your mental health:

Exercise often: It helps clear your mind and is great for your overall wellbeing

Talk to your friends: Ask them how they are doing; this will prompt them to ask you the same question. It's a great way to reach out if you are struggling to ask for help yourself.

Moderate alcohol: The best way to look after your mental health is with a clear head

Give back to others: It's amazing how awesome this simple task can make you feel

Find a hobby: It doesn't matter what it is, if you enjoy it keep doing it

Remember, you are number one, look after yourself first then you will be in a better position to help others!

Motivation

When looking for motivation find out what works for you. Ask yourself, how are you motivated? Is it intrinsically or extrinsically? Is it through positive reinforcement and self-talk or through negative feedback and comments? Once you've found out what works for you double down on it and go all in because motivation drives consistency and consistency is what get results!

A great way to stay motivated with your health and fitness goals is to use a wall calendar, you know, the ones you stick to the fridge or hang from the wall. Simply write at the bottom of the calendar the type of exercise you will do that month, for example, gym, yoga, swim, run, bike ride, tennis etc. Then once you have completed one of those exercise sessions just write it in the box. If however, you make it to the end of the day and didn't do any exercise then mark an X down. The aim of the game is to limit the number of Xs on the calendar each month.

It's such a great way to easily see how consistent you have been, plus you can see in advance if too many Xs are creeping in, which is your reminder to get out there and chalk up an exercise session. Remember when we talked about consistency being the key to getting results? Well this will sort that problem out no problem!

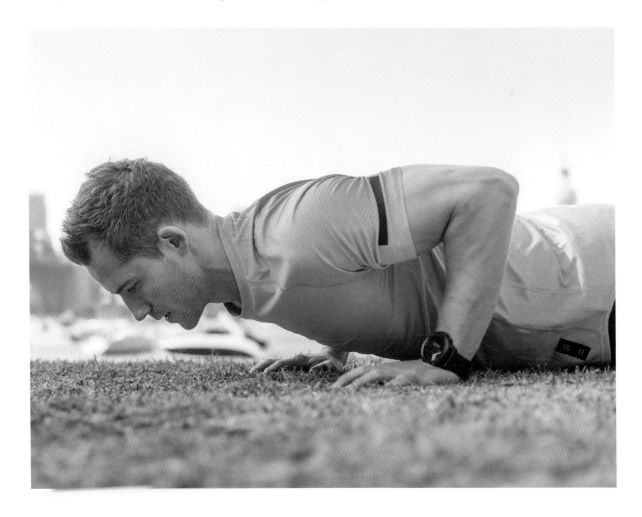

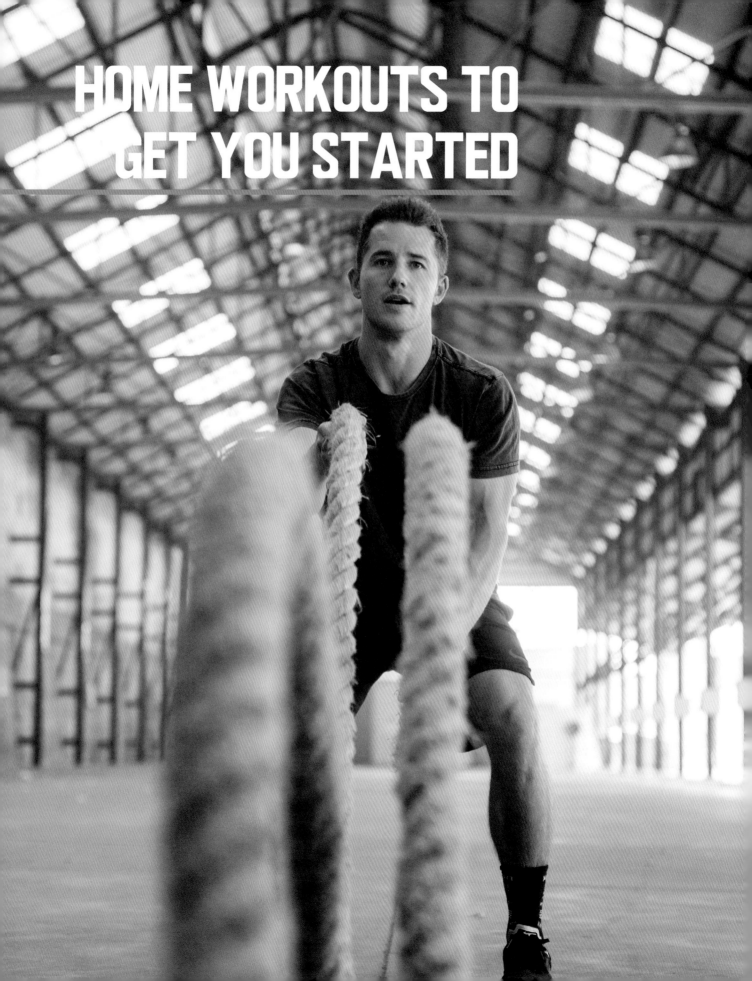

HOME WORKOUTS TO GET YOU STARTED

There are so many benefits with working out at home and you can absolutely work up a sweat, build strength and start crushing some serious calories in the process. Don't waste money on a gym membership if you don't like going to the gym. One of my rules when exercising is to choose a type of exercise you enjoy, and you can see yourself sticking to.

So fire up your fav playlist and get ready to move through some simple 20-minute exercise sessions that can be completed with minimal equipment.

To get started you will need:

an exercise or yoga mat

two dumbbells, two x 10–12 kg (22–26 lb) for men
and two x 7–10 kg (15–22 lb) for women

skipping rope

a medicine ball 8–10 kg (18–22 lb)

a Swiss ball (exercise ball)

Warming Up

Keep it simple. Have a look at the workout ahead and move through a few bodyweight versions of what's coming up in the workout e.g. bodyweight squats, push-ups, lunges etc. Just do so slowly and with care. Spending five minutes working through these exercises will help you to stay injury free and get your body ready for a great workout.

The Workouts

Once you have warmed up, set your timer for 20 minutes and get ready to hit that start button. When the workout starts to get tough, checking the timer to see you don't have long to go can be a great motivator.

Once you've chosen your workout level of beginner, intermediate or advanced, decide whether it's a strength session or a cardio session you'd like to work through.

Strength:

These sessions will help you to build muscle, prevent the risk of injury and make the aerobic or cardio sessions more productive. In order for the strength sessions to be effective look to overload the muscle by increasing the weight or slowing down the speed of the exercise, this will encourage your muscles to adapt, grow and get stronger. The numbers next to the **strength** exercises are the amount of repetitions to complete each time.

Cardio/Aerobic:

These sessions will help to improve your cardiovascular health, help with sleep, strengthen your immune system and boost your mood. HIIT or High Intensity Interval Training is a very effective way to **crush calories** and awesome if you're struggling for time but it's only effective if you work close to maximum intensity, meaning you must make every effort to push all the way through the rounds and complete as many repetitions as you can in the allotted time. If you are doing this correctly you should find this style of exercise extremely challenging.

Of course, if you want to double up on any of the sessions (making them last for 40 minutes) then go for it. You could mix and match a strength and cardio session together for the ultimate full-body burner. Remember there are plenty of ways to exercise, just make sure you are moving your body every day while doing something you enjoy.

OK, ready? Let's get moving!!!

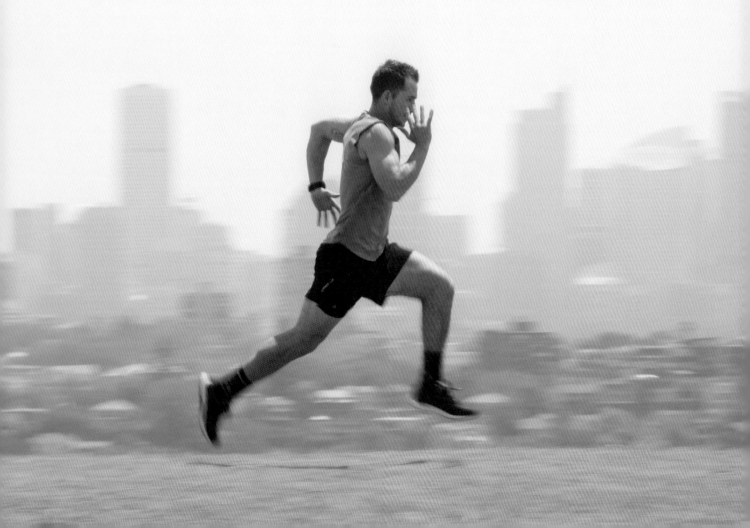

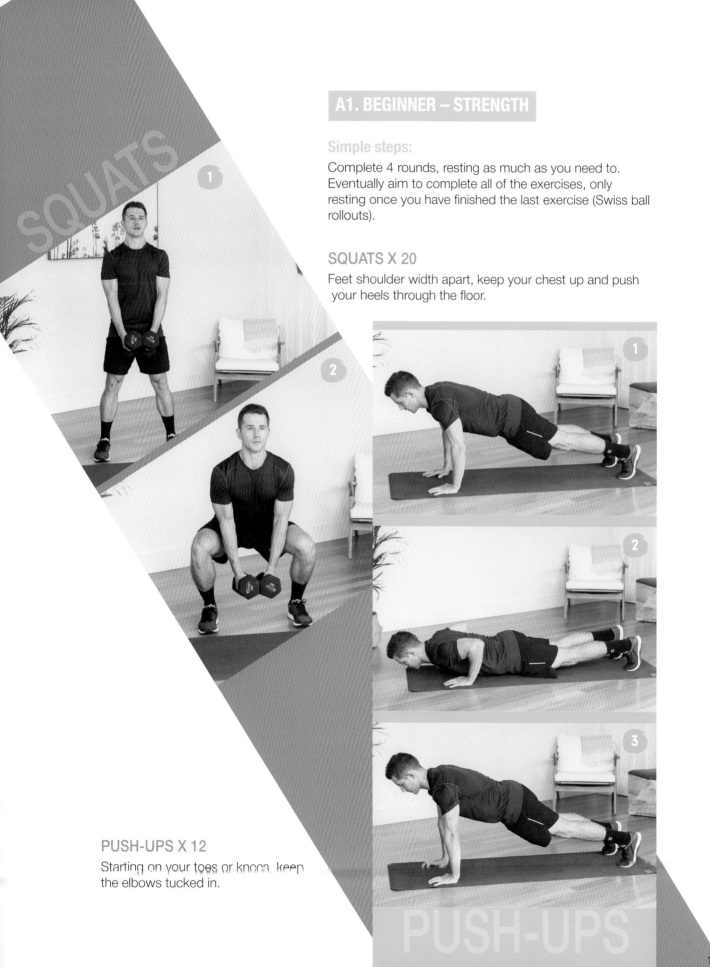

SQUATS

A1. BEGINNER – STRENGTH

Simple steps:

Complete 4 rounds, resting as much as you need to. Eventually aim to complete all of the exercises, only resting once you have finished the last exercise (Swiss ball rollouts).

SQUATS X 20

Feet shoulder width apart, keep your chest up and push your heels through the floor.

PUSH-UPS X 12

Starting on your toes or knees, keep the elbows tucked in.

PUSH-UPS

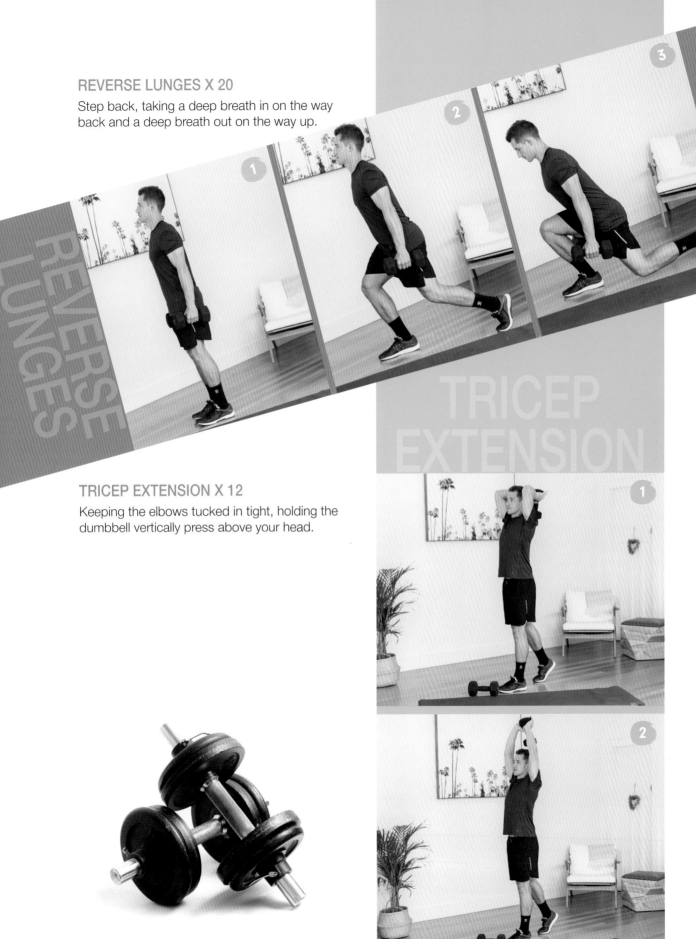

REVERSE LUNGES X 20

Step back, taking a deep breath in on the way back and a deep breath out on the way up.

TRICEP EXTENSION X 12

Keeping the elbows tucked in tight, holding the dumbbell vertically press above your head.

REVERSE LUNGES

TRICEP EXTENSION

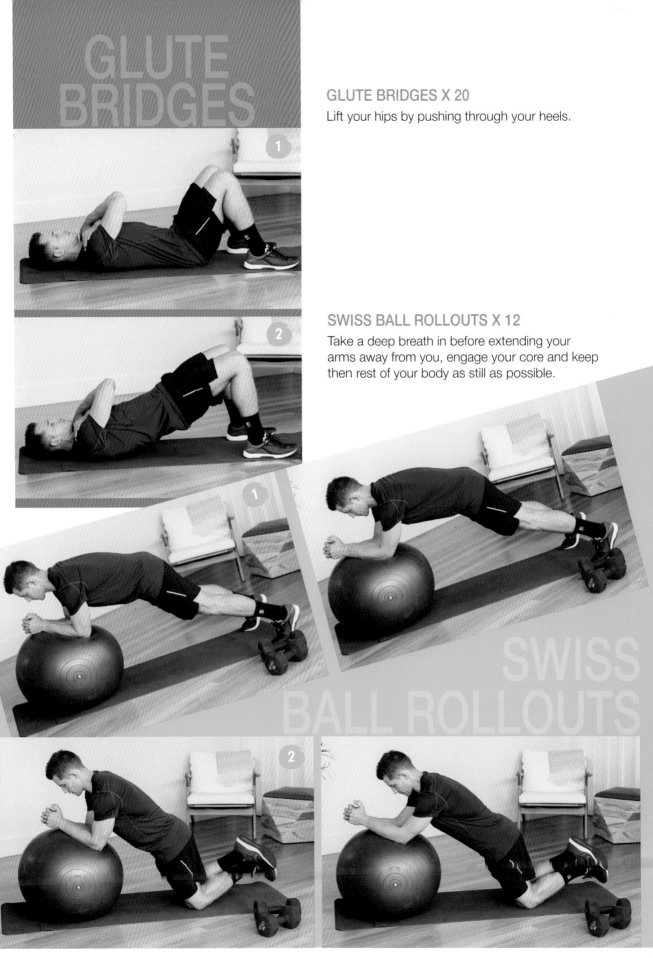

GLUTE BRIDGES

GLUTE BRIDGES X 20

Lift your hips by pushing through your heels.

SWISS BALL ROLLOUTS X 12

Take a deep breath in before extending your arms away from you, engage your core and keep then rest of your body as still as possible.

SWISS BALL ROLLOUTS

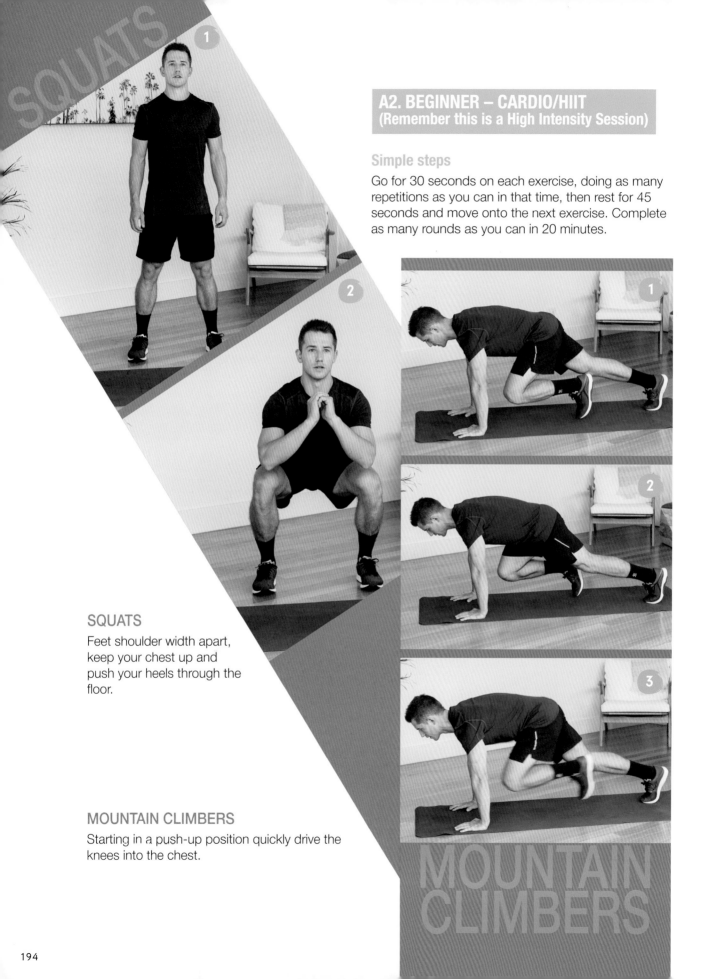

SQUATS

A2. BEGINNER – CARDIO/HIIT
(Remember this is a High Intensity Session)

Simple steps

Go for 30 seconds on each exercise, doing as many repetitions as you can in that time, then rest for 45 seconds and move onto the next exercise. Complete as many rounds as you can in 20 minutes.

SQUATS

Feet shoulder width apart, keep your chest up and push your heels through the floor.

MOUNTAIN CLIMBERS

Starting in a push-up position quickly drive the knees into the chest.

MOUNTAIN CLIMBERS

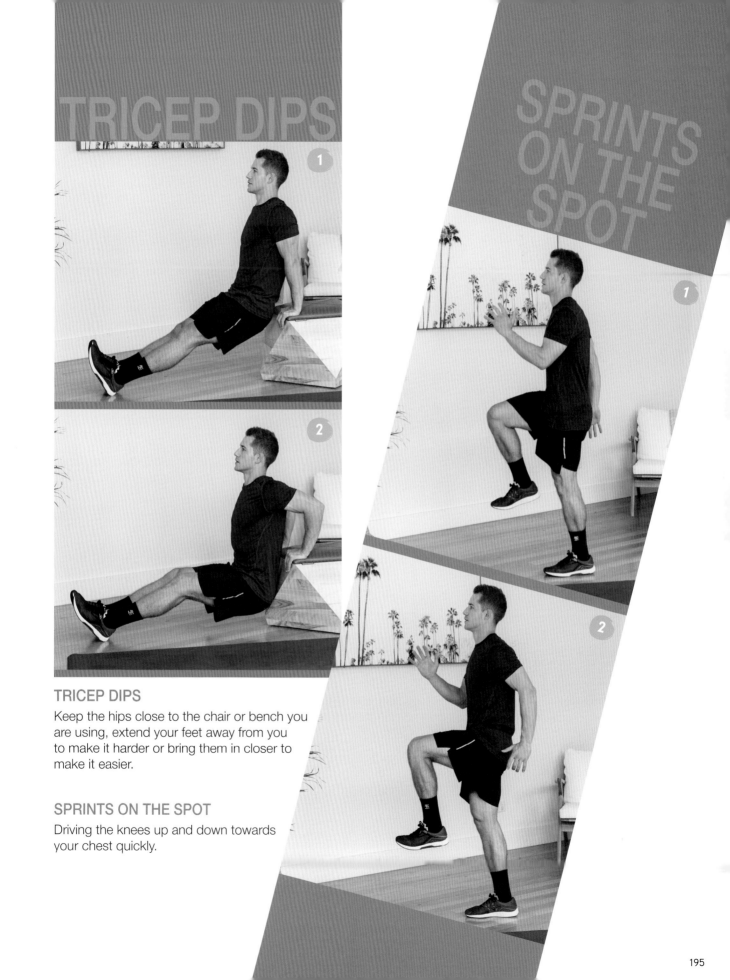

TRICEP DIPS

Keep the hips close to the chair or bench you are using, extend your feet away from you to make it harder or bring them in closer to make it easier.

SPRINTS ON THE SPOT

Driving the knees up and down towards your chest quickly.

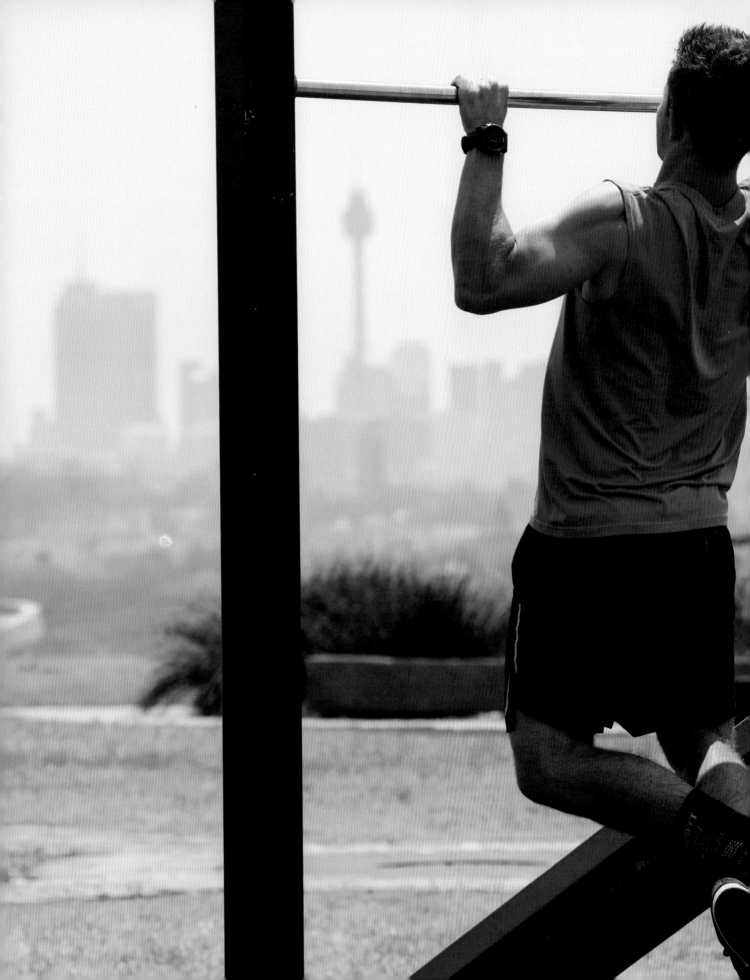

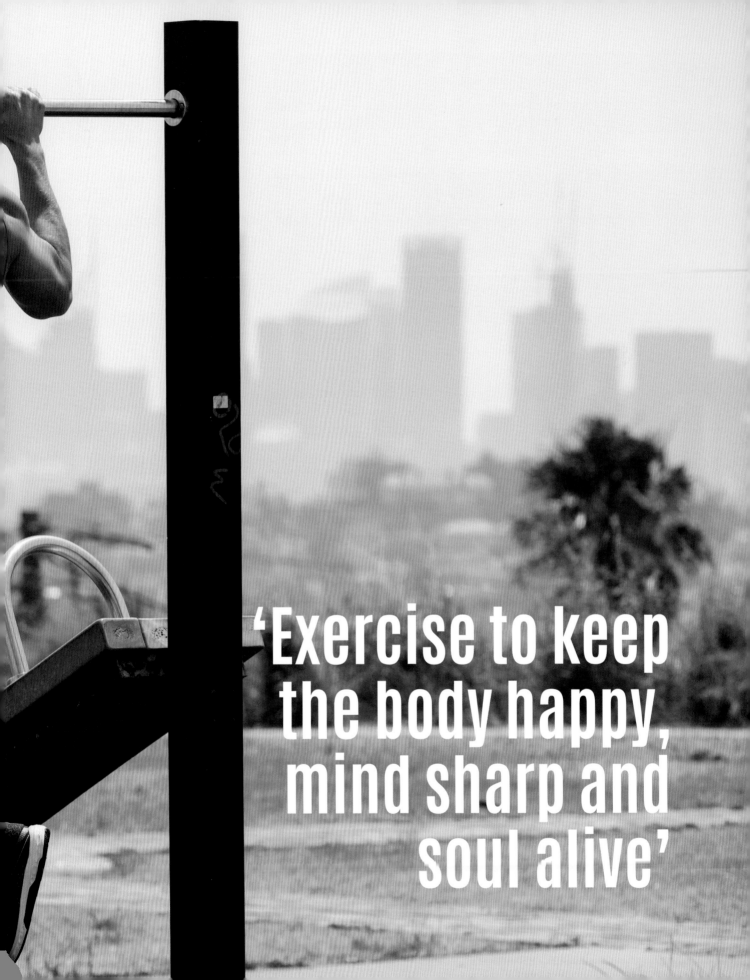

'Exercise to keep the body happy, mind sharp and soul alive'

CONTROLLED BICYCLE CRUNCHES

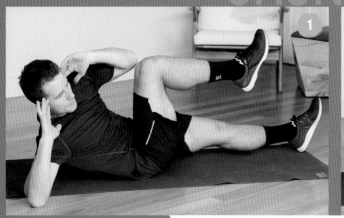

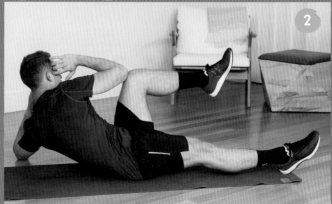

WALL SQUATS

CONTROLLED BICYCLE CRUNCHES

Bring your opposite elbow and knee towards each other slowly then repeat with the other side.

WALL SQUAT HOLD

Keep your shoulders back against the wall and hips level with the knees.

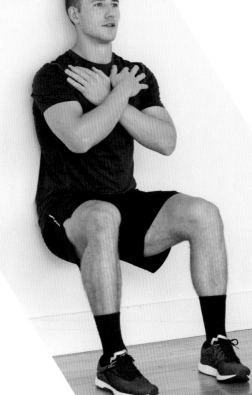

B1. INTERMEDIATE – STRENGTH

Simple steps:

Complete 4 rounds, resting as much as you need to. Eventually aim to complete all of the exercises only resting once you have finished the last exercise (supine crunches).

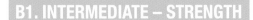

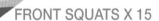

FRONT SQUATS X 15

Hold the dumbbell across your chest (use 2 if you're strong enough) push your heels through the floor.

SHOULDER PRESS X 12

Take a deep breath in as you lower the dumbbells, then breathe out as you push them away from you.

SHOULDER PRESS

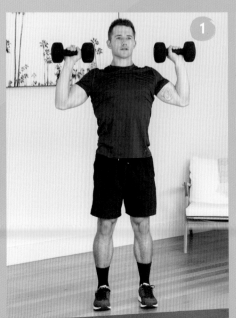

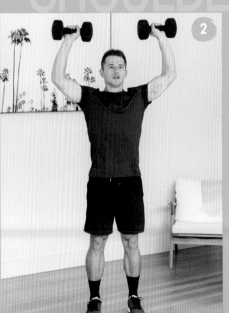

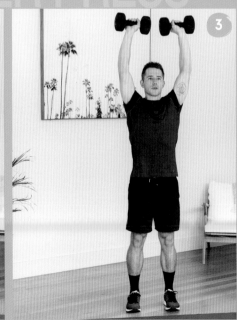

(BULGARIAN) SPLIT LEG SQUATS
X 10 EACH LEG

Resting your back leg on a chair or low bench, bend your front leg lowering yourself to the ground slowly, engage your core and slowly squeeze your quad and glute as you stand back up. At the top of the rep keep the knee slightly bent.

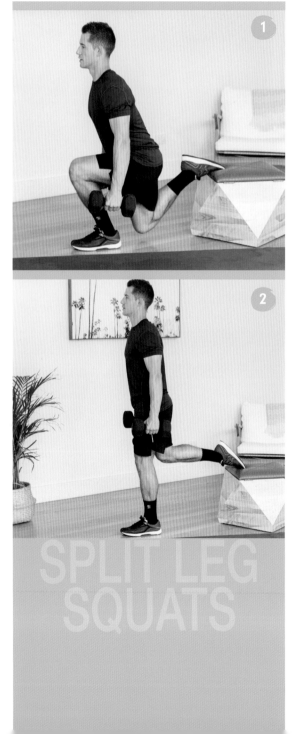

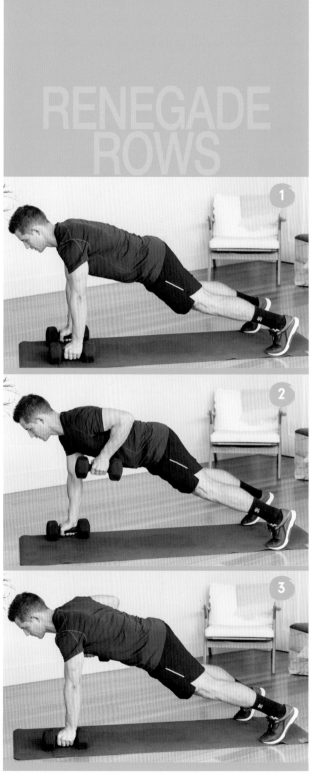

RENEGADE ROWS X 12

Starting in a push-up position holding the dumbbells, slowly lift one at a time into the chest then lowering them back down. Keep your hips as still as possible.

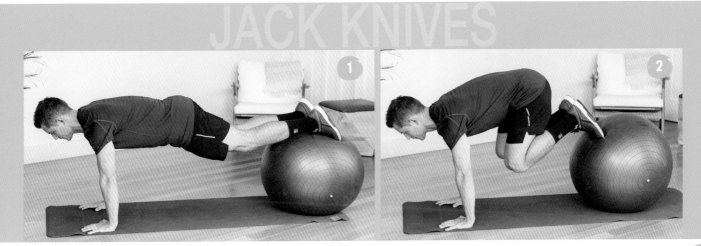

JACK KNIVES X 12

Resting your feet on the Swiss ball, pull your knees into your chest while lifting your hips a little.

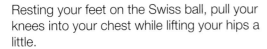

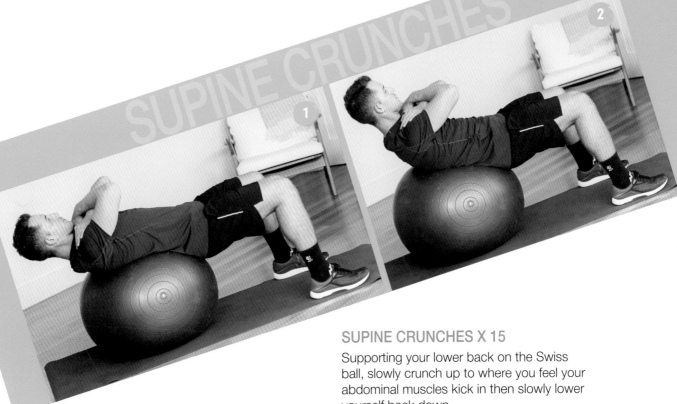

SUPINE CRUNCHES X 15

Supporting your lower back on the Swiss ball, slowly crunch up to where you feel your abdominal muscles kick in then slowly lower yourself back down.

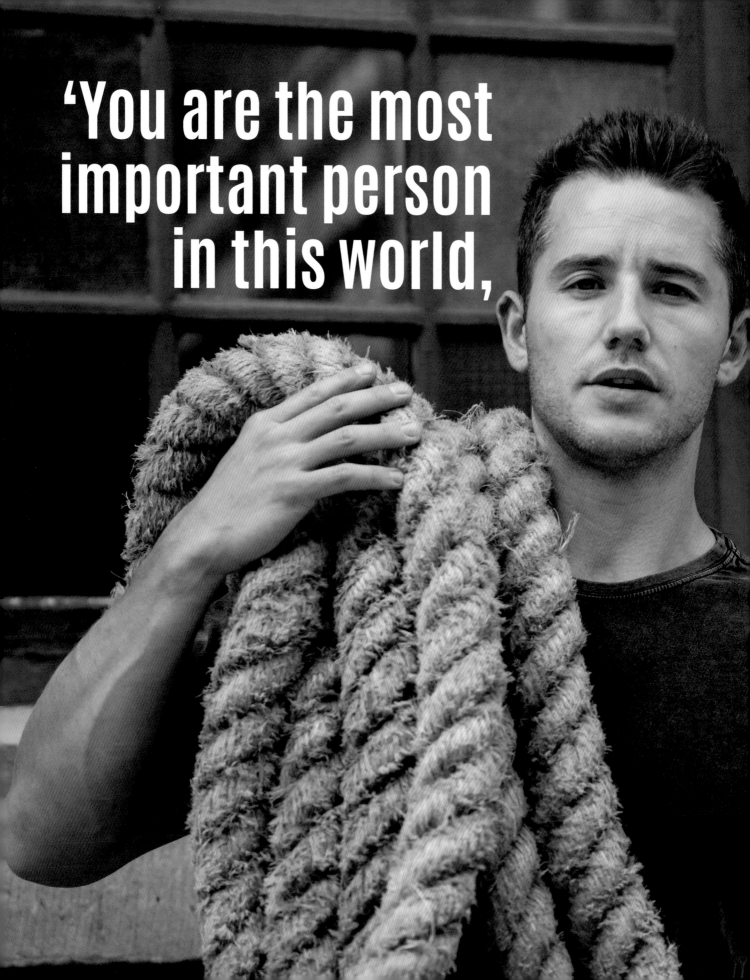

'You are the most important person in this world,

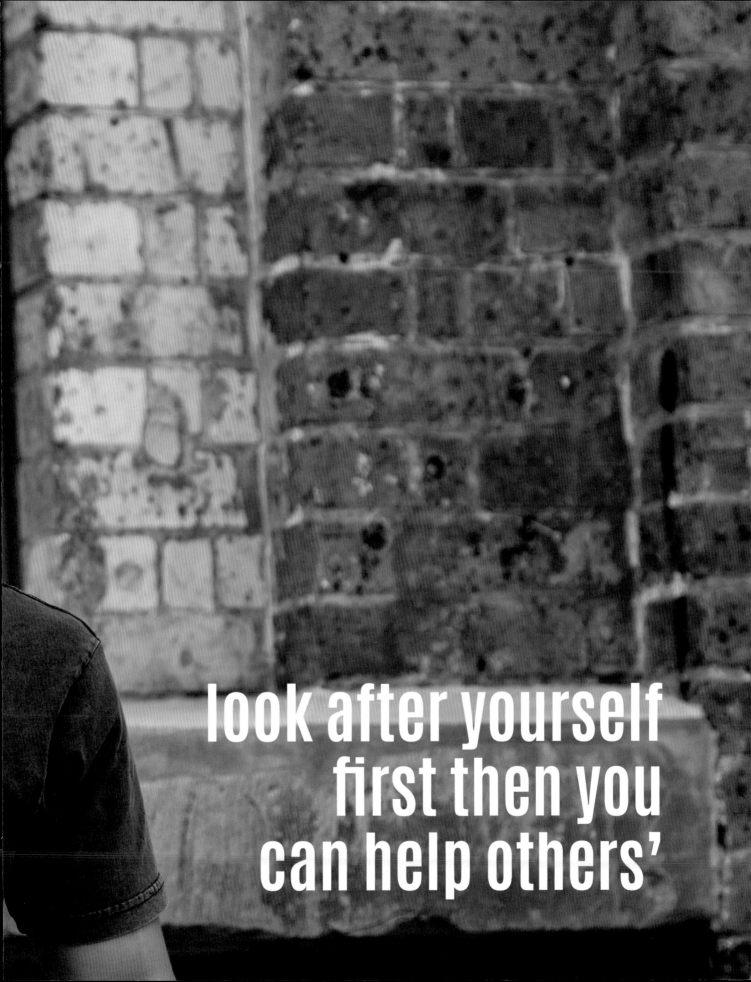

look after yourself
first then you
can help others'

B2. INTERMEDIATE – CARDIO/HIIT
(Remember this is a High Intensity Session)

Simple steps:

Go for 30 seconds on each exercise, doing as many repetitions as you can in that time, then rest for 30 seconds and move onto the next exercise. Complete as many rounds as you can in 20 minutes.

SKIPPING

Make big circles with your wrists and stay light on your feet.

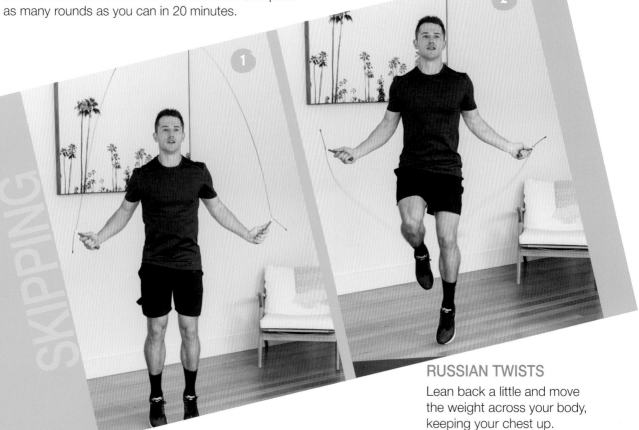

RUSSIAN TWISTS

Lean back a little and move the weight across your body, keeping your chest up.

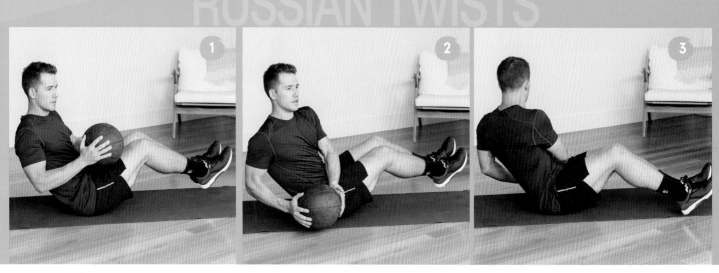

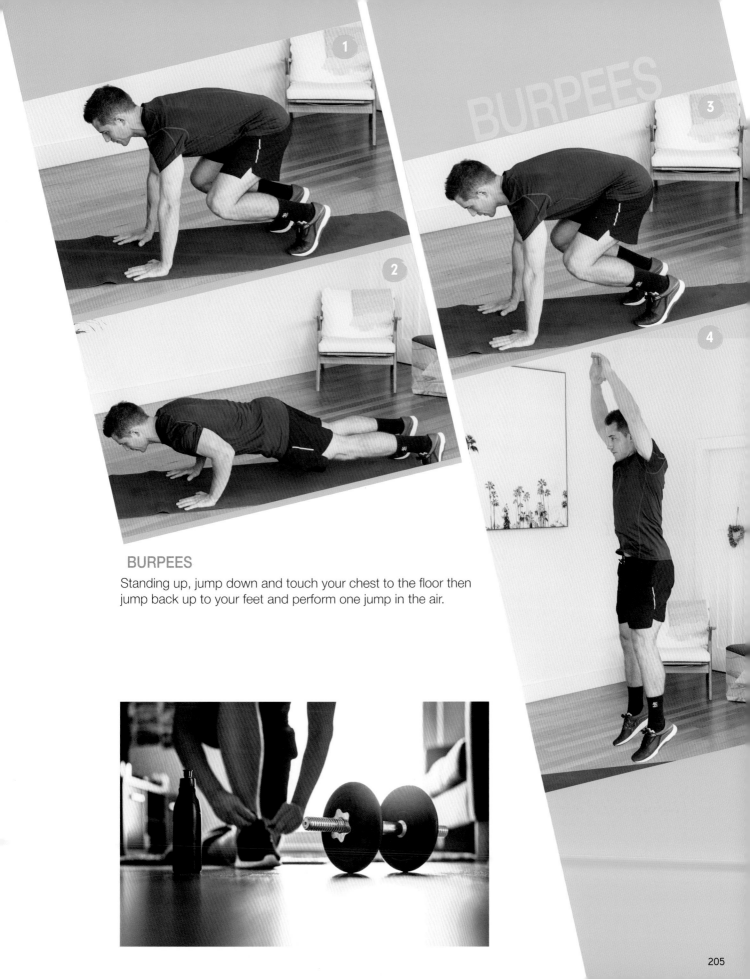

BURPEES

Standing up, jump down and touch your chest to the floor then jump back up to your feet and perform one jump in the air.

205

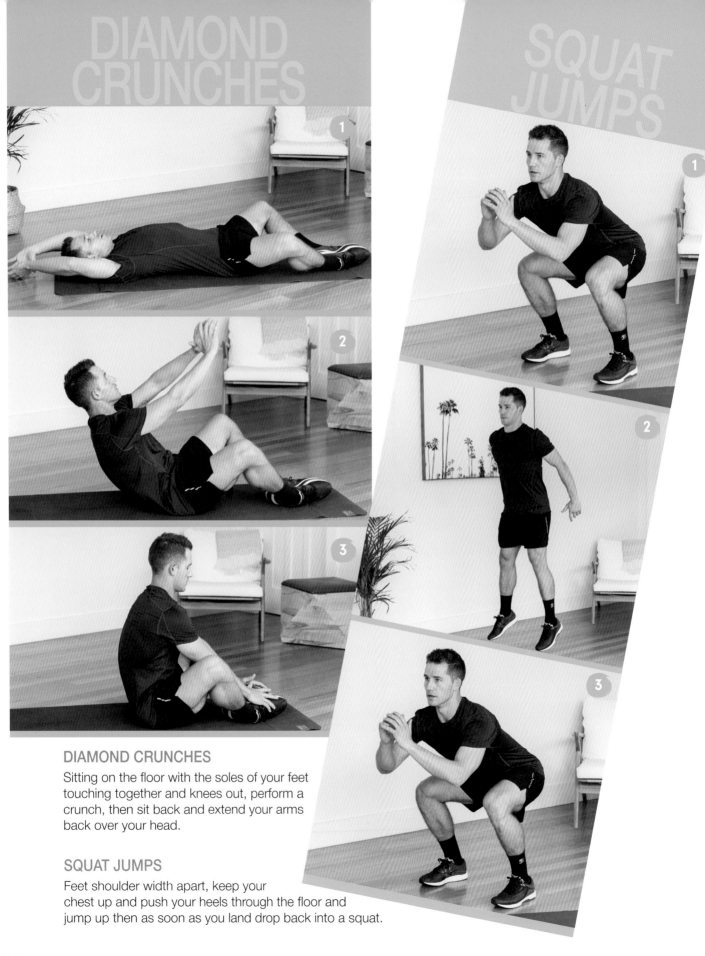

DIAMOND CRUNCHES

Sitting on the floor with the soles of your feet touching together and knees out, perform a crunch, then sit back and extend your arms back over your head.

SQUAT JUMPS

Feet shoulder width apart, keep your chest up and push your heels through the floor and jump up then as soon as you land drop back into a squat.

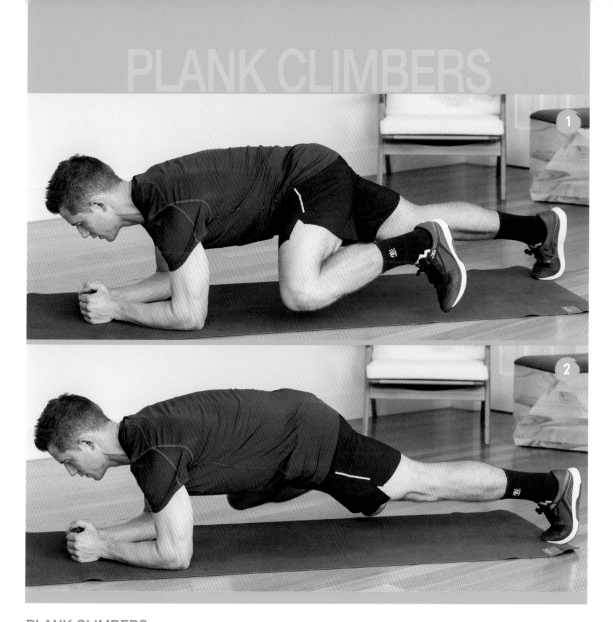

PLANK CLIMBERS

Start in a plank position, lift one knee up and to the side of your body, alternating each rep.

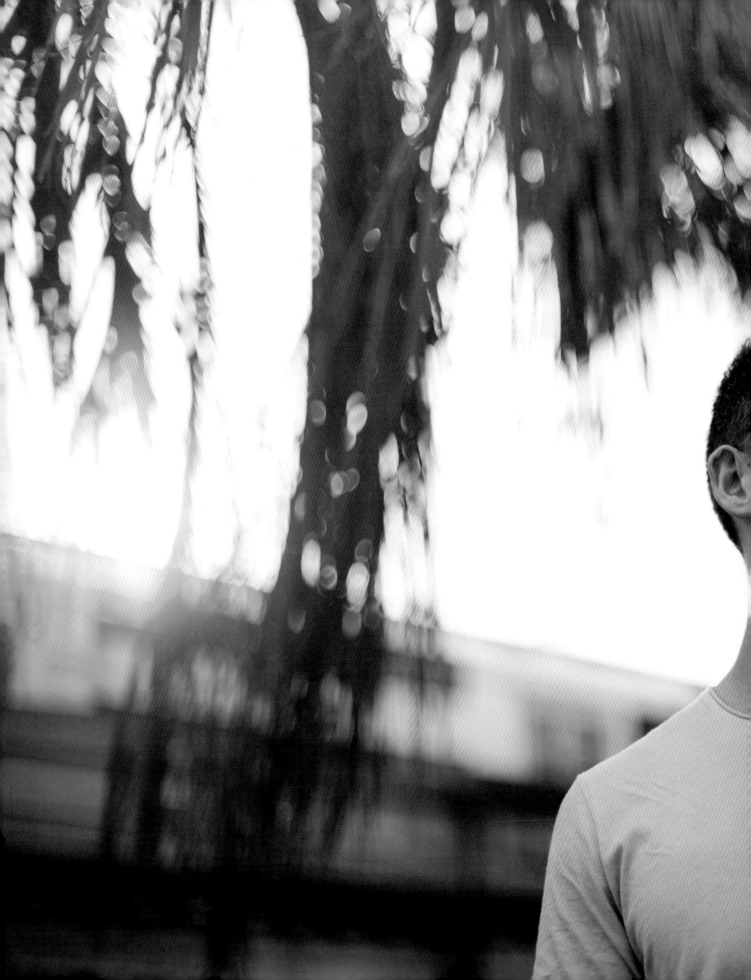

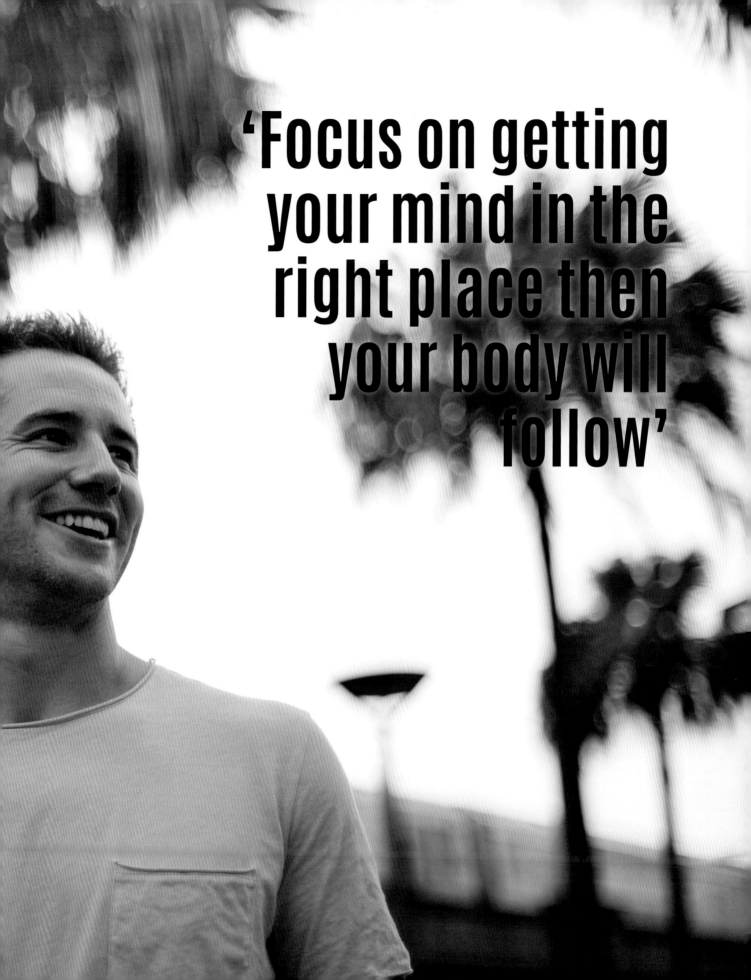

'Focus on getting your mind in the right place then your body will follow'

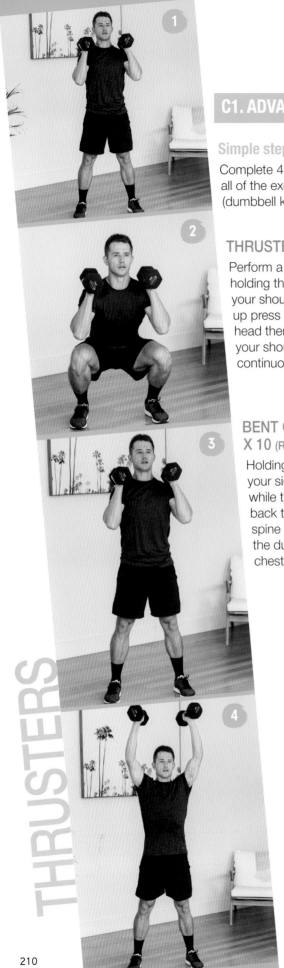

THRUSTERS

C1. ADVANCED – STRENGTH

Simple steps:

Complete 4 rounds, resting as much as you need to. Eventually aim to complete all of the exercises, only resting once you have finished the last exercise (dumbbell kick backs).

THRUSTERS X 10

Perform a squat while holding the dumbbells on your shoulders, as you stand up press them above your head then lower down to your shoulders and repeat continuously.

BENT OVER ROWS
X 10 (RIGHT)

Holding the dumbbells by your side, hinge forward while tilting your tailbone back to ensure your spine is straight. Pull the dumbbells into your chest slowly.

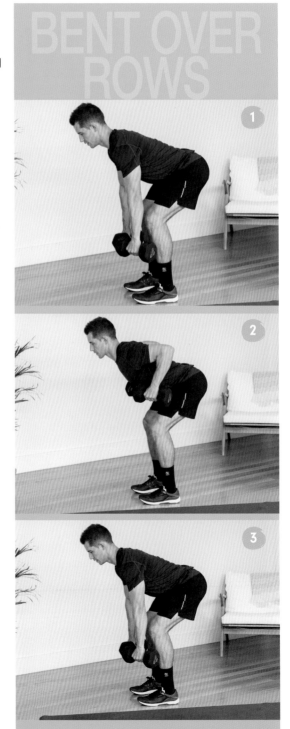

BENT OVER ROWS

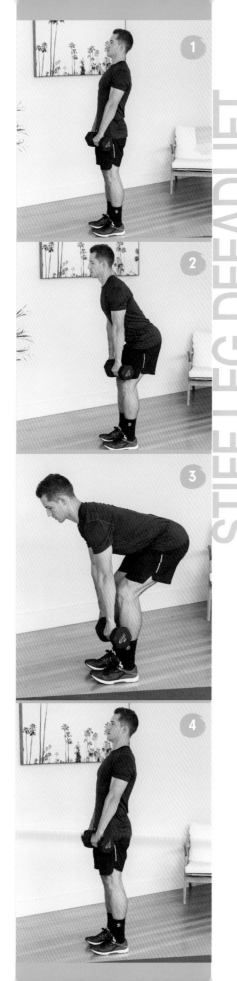

STIFF LEG DEADLIFT X 10

Stand with your feet a little narrower than shoulder width apart and holding the dumbbells in front of your thighs. Hinge forward while tilting your tailbone back. Slightly bend the knees but not too much and feel your hamstrings stretch, then stand up whilst all the time keeping your shoulders back.

Z-PRESS X 10

Sit up straight with your legs extended and chest proud, perform a slow, controlled shoulder press, keep your torso still and core engaged.

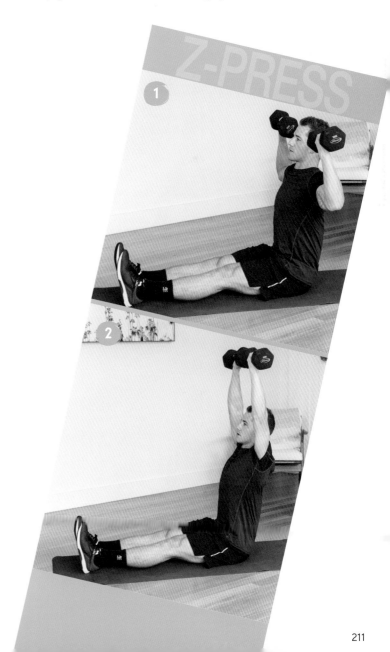

STEP BACK
LUNGE WITH
BICEP CURL

STEP BACK LUNGE WITH BICEP CURL X 10 EACH LEG

Holding the dumbbells by your side, as you step back perform a bicep curl then step back up and repeat with the opposite leg.

DOUBLE DUMBBELL KICK BACK X 10

Holding the dumbbells by your side, hinge forward while tilting your tailbone back. Bend the elbows and push the dumbbells backwards, when they reach in line with your back turn your palms up to the sky, forcing the triceps to work a little more.

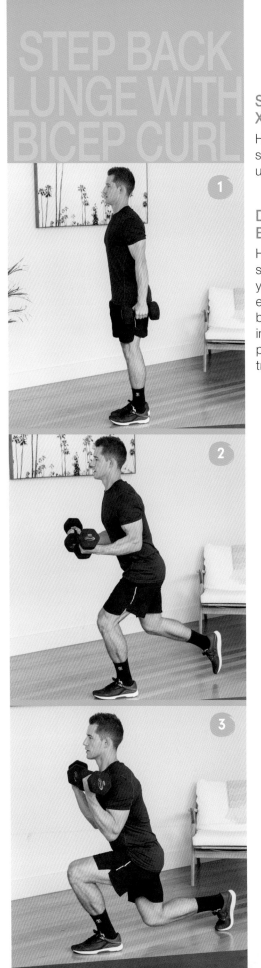

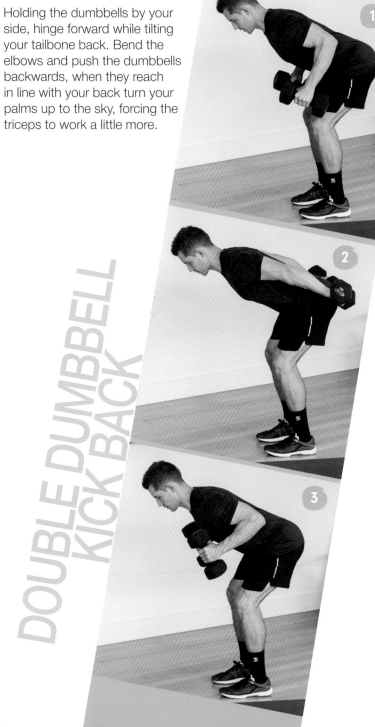

DOUBLE DUMBBELL
KICK BACK

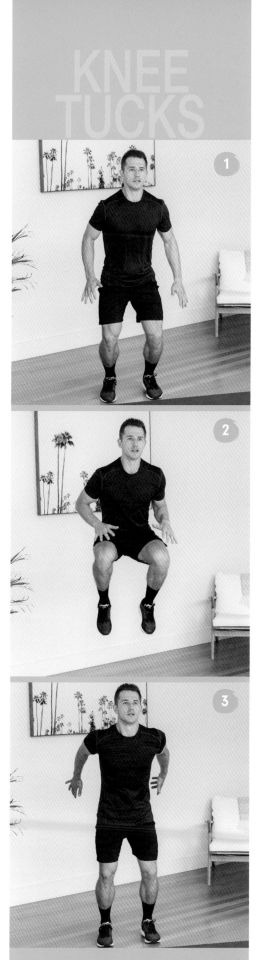

KNEE TUCKS

C2. ADVANCED – CARDIO/HIIT
(Remember this is a High Intensity Session)

Simple steps:

Go for 30 seconds on each exercise, doing as many repetitions as you can in that time, then rest for 20 seconds and move onto the next exercise. Complete as many rounds as you can in 20 minutes.

KNEE TUCKS

Starting with your feet shoulder width apart, jump up and tuck your knees into your chest, land softly and repeat.

PUSH-UPS AND CLIMBERS

Perform one push-up then 6 climbers, lifting your right then left knee into your chest quickly.

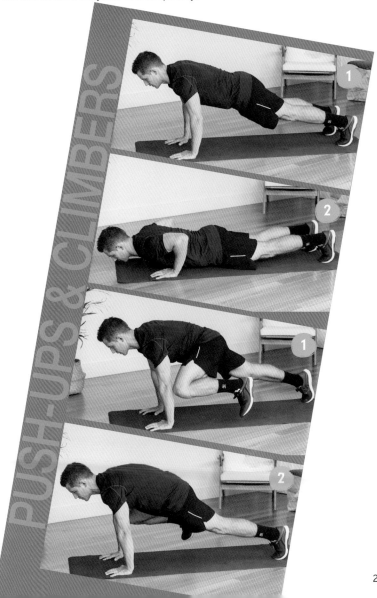

PUSH-UPS & CLIMBERS

JUMPING LUNGES

Start in a lunge, jump up and quickly switch feet in midair, as you land stay soft on your knees with your chest up. Use your arms and drive backwards and forwards.

SWISS BALL ROLL OUTS

Starting in a plank on the Swiss ball, slowly extend the arms away from you taking a deep breath in as you do this then breathing out as you bring them back into your body.

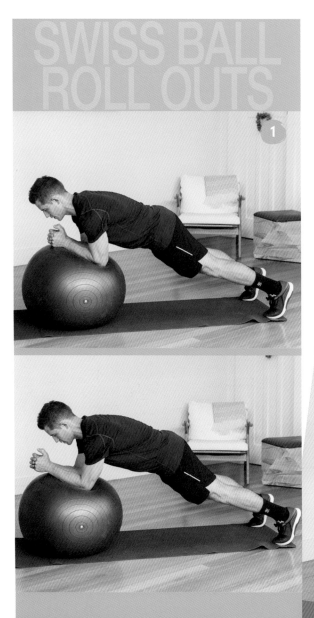

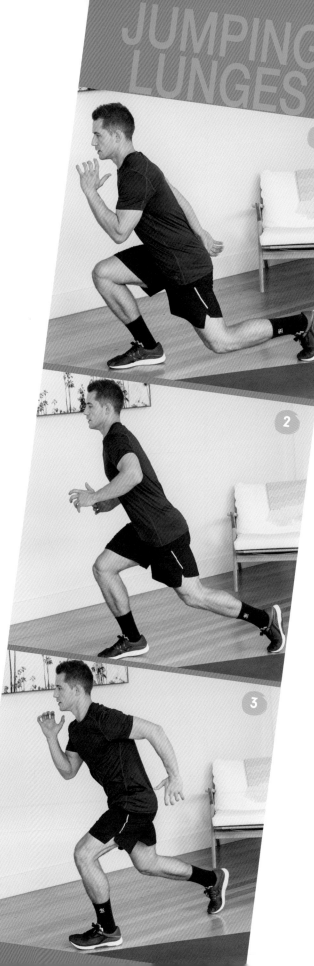

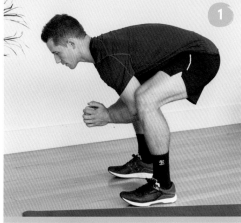

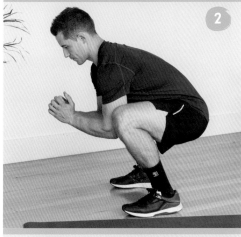

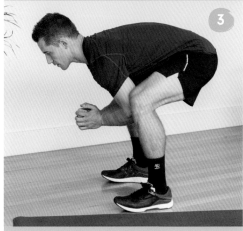

FROG SQUATS

Set up in a deep squat with your elbows positioned on the inside of your thighs, lift your hips then drop them back down quickly and repeat. You will feel your quads working instantly.

HALF HINDUS

Start with your hands on the floor, weight on your toes and bum high in the air. Drop your chest to the floor dipping down low then arching your back and lifting your chest up and extending through your arms. Repeat in reverse finishing with your hips high.

HALF HINDUS

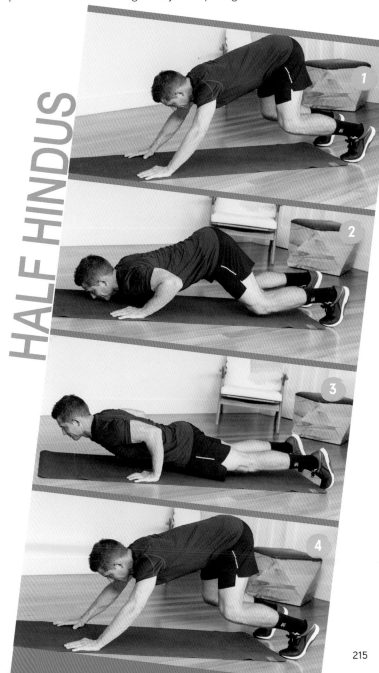

ACKNOWLEDGEMENTS

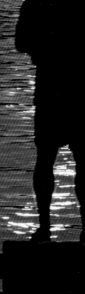

If you had said to me 16 years ago, while I was sitting in a classroom about to take my English exams, that one day I would be using what I had learnt to help me write my very own health and fitness cookbook I would have laughed at you and said absolutely no way. But now this has actually happened and I'm so proud of what I have achieved.

My goal when I first became qualified in the health and fitness industry over 10 years ago was to simplify people's approach to exercise and nutrition and I really believe this book does just that.

A lot of blood, sweat and tears have gone into creating this book and I owe it all to three people: Kieron, Christian and Gareth. You have believed, supported and trusted in me since day one. You're mentors, friends and everything I have achieved is because you have been behind me. You've taught me that hard work and dedication is the key to success in anything you do. Boys, thank you for believing in me.

To my fiancée Elle, thank you for just being you and for always supporting and allowing me to pursue my passion in life. I'm sorry for the mess I always leave in the kitchen after recipe testing late at night! I do try to keep the food off the floor and on the chopping board, honestly …

To my mum Jane, who taught me everything I know about cooking. Your recipes aren't always super healthy, but they are always super delicious. I'll never forget standing on the chair in our kitchen at home at just six years old learning how to chop, bake and create delicious food with you. It was these moments that made me realize I loved not only eating food but also learning how to make it.

To Fiona Schultz and all of the team at New Holland Publishers. Thank you for giving me this chance to write my first book – hopefully this is the start of something very special together.

To Steven McArthur and Natasha Rontziokos at Buzz Group, who have worked tirelessly to get this into production, thank you. We make a great team.

Finally, to my sister Chloë, her husband Chris and my little niece Isla. Having you all so close by is very special and being able to cook for you all on Sunday night reminds me of growing up and remembering how food brought us together, to chat, to laugh and to tell stories. Isla, I'm looking forward to passing on what Granny Jane taught me so you too can learn one of life's great skills – cooking!

Rich :)

Index Recipes

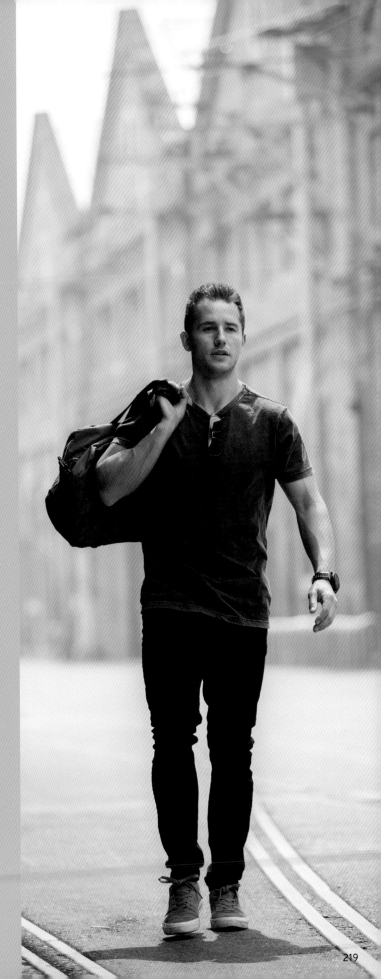

Index Exercises

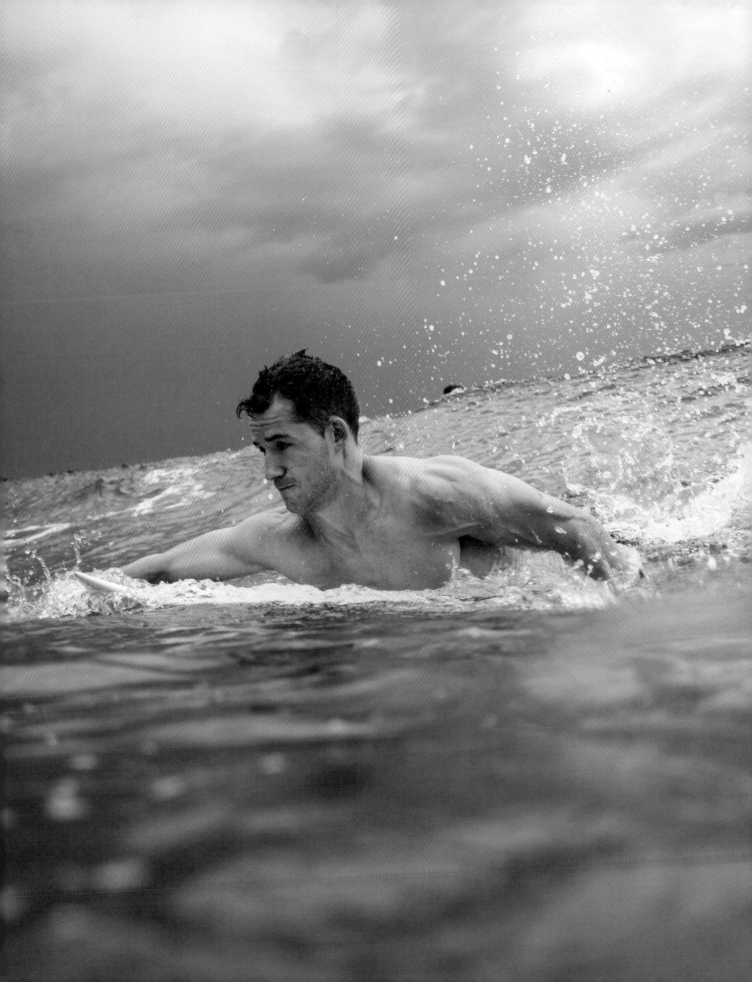

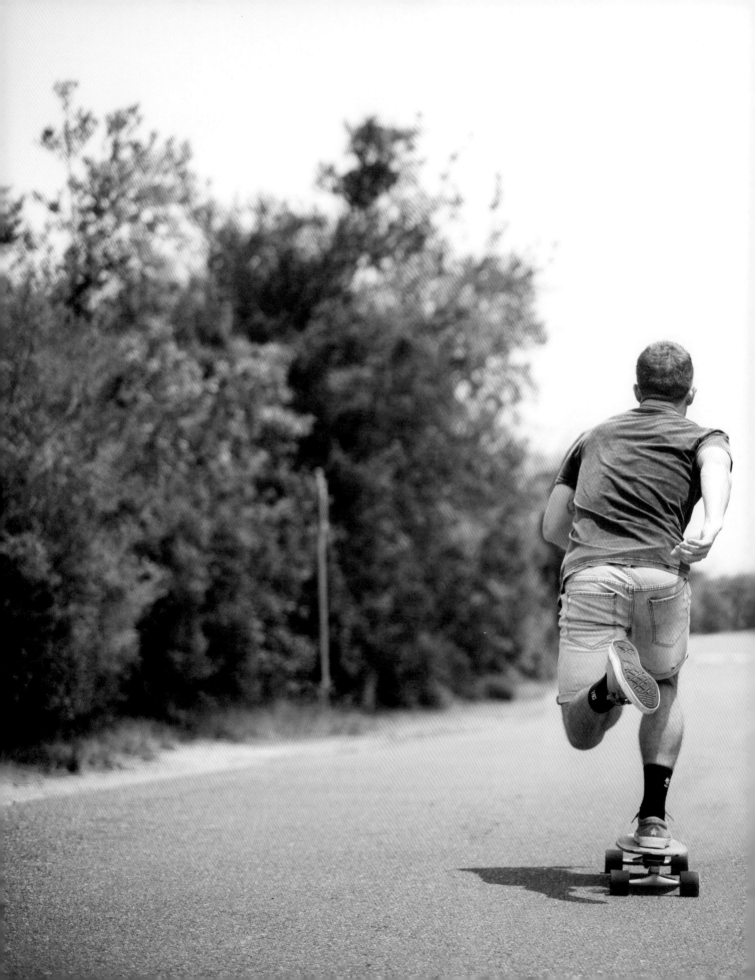

'keep it simple and play the long game of health'

First published in 2021 by New Holland Publishers
Sydney • Auckland

Level 1, 178 Fox Valley Road, Wahroonga 2076, Australia
5/39 Woodside Ave, Northcote, Auckland 0627, New Zealand
newhollandpublishers.com

Copyright © 2021 New Holland Publishers
Copyright © 2021 in text: Richard Kerrign
Copyright © 2021 in images: Fitness and Lifestyle - Remy Brand,
Recipes - Rob Palmer

A record of this book is held at the National Library of Australia.

ISBN 9781760792589

Group Managing Director: Fiona Schultz
Publisher: Fiona Schultz
Project Editor: Liz Hardy
Designer: Yolanda La Gorcé
Stylist: Kristina Jackson
Production Director: Arlene Gippert

Printed in China

10 9 8 7 6 5 4 3 2 1

Keep up with New Holland Publishers:
NewHollandPublishers
@newhollandpublishers

$30.00 US